Coping With Sports Injuries: Psychological strategies for rehabilitation

Jane Crossman,

School of Kinesiology,
Lakehead University,
Canada

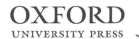

OXFORD

UNIVERSITY PRESS

itally and produced in a standard specification
sure its continuing availability

OXFORD
UNIVERSITY PRESS

Great Clarendon Street, Oxford OX2 6DP

Oxford University Press is a department of the University of Oxford.
It furthers the University's objective of excellence in research, scholarship,
and education by publishing worldwide in

Oxford New York

Auckland   Cape Town Dar es Salaam Hong Kong   Karachi
Kuala Lumpur Madrid Melbourne Mexico City Nairobi
New Delhi Shanghai Taipei Toronto
With offices in
Argentina Austria Brazil Chile Czech Republic France Greece
Guatemala Hungary Italy Japan South Korea Poland Portugal
Singapore Switzerland Thailand Turkey Ukraine Vietnam

Oxford is a registered trade mark of Oxford University Press
in the UK and in certain other countries

Published in the United States
by Oxford University Press Inc., New York

Oxford is a registered trade mark of Oxford University Press
in the UK and in certain other countries

Published in the United States
by Oxford University Press Inc., New York

© Oxford University Press 2001

ISBN 0-19-263215-9

Preface

Wherever I've travelled in the world, physicians specializing in sports medicine, physiotherapists, and sports therapists have told me that they realize that helping athletes recover from injury involves more than just physical rehabilitation. They've also told me repeatedly that they want and need to know more about how psychological variables interplay with physical healing. Moreover, they want to be able to incorporate the 'psychological side' of rehabilitation into their practice. As a researcher in this area, I was acutely aware that there was a need for a practical book for medical practitioners that addressed psychological issues. Thus, *Coping With Sports Injuries: Psychological strategies for rehabilitation* was born.

Medical practitioners are in an excellent position to identify athletes who are not coping well with their injury. The attitude of medical practitioners towards the injury and the manner in which they respond and communicate to their clients can have a profound influence on how athletes view their injury and subsequent rehabilitation. Although this book has been written primarily for medical practitioners, the contents could well be of value to others in the sport community, such as coaches and athletes.

The primary authors of each chapter are some of the world's leading researchers and authorities concerning the psychological dynamics influencing sport injury. They were chosen not only because of their impressive publication records and hands-on experience working with injured athletes, but because they possessed specific expertise in the topics which I deemed were important to include.

While designing the content of this book, I was mindful of the need to address the issues that medical practitioners have told me they want to know more about. We (the contributors) hope to have achieved this in a useful, comprehensive, cohesive, and reader-friendly book. As the editor, I've tried to eliminate unnecessary overlap and inconsistencies of material.

I feel confident in stating that the information provided in this book is the most up-to-date possible. Because the sequencing of chapters has been purposely coordinated, it is recommended that the ten chapters be read in consecutive order. However, because the chapters are so distinctive in their content, it is possible to consult chapters in random order.

In Chapter 1, Britt Brewer examines the emotional reactions that athletes may experience following the onset of injury. Physicians, physiotherapists, and sport therapists working in clinical settings often observe that negative emotions experienced as a result of injury can influence the athlete's attitude toward, and subsequent recovery from injury. This chapter provides an overview of issues associated with the emotional adjustment of athletes to injury. Strategies for recognizing poor emotional adjustment and ways to improve it are also discussed.

In Chapter 2, Aynsley Smith and colleagues provide guidelines for assessing the psychosocial aspects of injury. Frequently used questionnaires are described and samples provided, as are ways to accurately interpret findings. The authors also provide guidelines for conducting the assessment interview.

Drawing upon his experience as a physician specializing in sports medicine and a former Olympian, David Gerrard, in Chapter 3, examines the role of the physician. The importance of entwining physical and psychological rehabilitation is emphasized.

Following on from this, Sandy Gordon and colleagues discuss the roles and responsibilities of physiotherapists and sport therapists in the rehabilitative process. Ways in which they can help the athlete adjust during recovery are also covered. The effective use of mental skills' techniques within the rehabilitation context is illustrated in three case studies.

In Chapter 5, Gretchen Kerr and Patricia Miller discuss the various ways that injured athletes cope with their injury. Mediating factors—such as the severity of the injury, the point in the competitive season at which the athlete was injured, and the type of injury—affect the choice and efficacy of various coping strategies. Such factors are explored in this chapter.

Medical practitioners sometimes erroneously assume that their clients adhere or comply with their rehabilitation regime. Low adherence and poor compliance are factors limiting effective recovery. Therefore, in Chapter 6, Adrian Taylor and Caroline Marlow describe strategies to increase compliance. Included in their discussion is the importance of changing predisposing factors and engaging the athlete in ownership of the rehabilitation program, as well as other strategies proven to improve compliance, such as goal-setting and effective communication.

In Chapter 7, I provide the tools to assist medical practitioners in helping injured athletes to think positively, manage stress effectively, and control pain via non-pharmacological techniques. Also, I provide guidelines for using strategies to enhance healing and control pain such as relaxation, imagery, autogenic training, and systematic desensitization.

The point is clearly made by Eileen Udry in Chapter 8 that successful recovery requires the social support of the athlete's coach, family, and teammates. The author discusses the role of these three support providers, as well as their effects on the postinjury status of the athlete. Finally, practical strategies of working and communicating with injured athletes' significant others are discussed.

In the penultimate chapter, Mark Andersen explores the process of returning to action and preventing future injury. The decision regarding when to return may be clouded by a profound desire of the athlete, coach, significant others, or a combination thereof, to get back to action as soon as possible; consequently, the return may be premature. Issues that may complicate the return, such as eating disorders and anxiety, are also discussed.

In the final chapter, David Gilbourne provides guidelines for integrating change into the workplace. It is hoped that the preceding chapters will have motivated you to want to make changes in your practice. This chapter provides you with the tools with which to make these changes through the process of systematic reflection and action research. A case study is provided as a means of illustrating the various steps involved in workplace change.

In summary, this book represents an attempt to integrate the work of some of the world's leading authorities in order to develop a comprehensive understanding of the psychological factors that affect success in the recovery from a sport injury.

All the people I initially contacted to participate in this project were willing to become involved, and to them I owe a great deal of thanks for their willingness to share their expertise. I also am very grateful to Chris Wreszczak for her invaluable assistance in the preparation of this manuscript.

J.C.

Ontario, Canada

November 2000

Contents

About the contributors

Dr Mark B. Andersen is a registered psychologist and Associate Professor at Victoria University in Melbourne, Australia. He received his doctorate from the University of Arizona in 1988 and immigrated to Australia in 1994. His teaching includes statistics, research design, rehabilitation psychology, and the professional practise of psychology. His research interests include the psychology of injury and rehabilitation; the role of exercise in mental health, well-being, and quality of life; the training and supervision of graduate students; and sport psychology service delivery. He is the first and current editor of the Professional Practice section of the international journal *The Sport Psychologist*.

Dr Britton W. Brewer is an Associate Professor of Psychology at Springfield College in Springfield, Massachusetts, USA, where he teaches undergraduate and graduate psychology courses, conducts research on psychological aspects of sport injury, and coaches the men's cross-country team. He received his doctorate in psychology (clinical) from Arizona State University in 1991. He is listed in the United States Olympic Committee Sport Psychology Registry, 1996–2000, and is a Certified Consultant to the Association for the Advancement of Applied Sport Psychology.

Dr Jane Crossman is a Professor of Kinesiology at Lakehead University in Thunder Bay, Ontario, Canada, where she teaches the sociology of sport, mental training, and research methods and was Chair for 6 years. She is an Associate Editor of *The Journal of Sport Behavior* and frequently reviews texts and other academic publications. Jane has helped elite athletes with their mental preparation in cycling, alpine skiing, curling, ski jumping, running, and swimming. She's a Fellow of the Association for the Advancement of Applied Sport Psychology and a member of the Canadian Mental Training Registry. During sabbatical leaves, Jane has been a Visiting Professor at the Universities of Exeter and Brighton (UK) and the University of Otago (New Zealand).

Nicole Detling was a Johannson–Gund Research Scholar at the Mayo Clinic Sports Medicine Center, USA, where she worked on a variety of psychophysiological, performance enhancement and injury-related research projects. She is pursuing her doctoral degree at the University of Utah in sport psychology. She has presented at several sport psychology conferences and has co-authored several manuscripts. She has conducted research in the area of physical and psychosocial outcome of injury and, thus, has worked with injured athletes regarding the psychosocial effects of injury. She has served as the performance enhancement consultant with coaches, athletes, and teams from the youth to the elite levels.

Dr David Gerrard is Associate Professor of Sports Medicine and Associate Dean at the University of Otago Medical School, Dunedin, New Zealand. He is a consultant sports physician with research interests in paediatric sports medicine, injury prevention, and the bioethics of medicine in sport. He is a member of the FINA Medical Committee and has had a long involvement in Olympic sport as an athlete (1964), NZ Team Physician (1984 and 1988) and NZ Team *Chef de Mission* in Atlanta (1996). As an athlete he is a former Olympic swimming semifinalist (Tokyo 1964) and a Commonwealth Games gold medallist in butterfly (Kingston 1966). In 1995, David was awarded The Order of the British Empire (OBE) for his contribution to medicine and sport.

Dr David Gilbourne is currently a principal lecturer in sport psychology and qualitative research methods at Liverpool John Moores University, UK. After qualifying as a teacher of physical education, he received his BA.and MSc degrees from The University of North East London and was awarded his PhD from the University of Brighton. In a professional context, he is accredited by the British Association for Sport and Exercise Sciences as both an applied psychologist and researcher. His research interests include the application of action research within sports settings and the exploration of alternative forms of representation through the mediums of life story and life history.

Dr Sandy Gordon is Senior Lecturer in the Department of Human Movement and Exercise Science at The University of Western Australia, where he teaches undergraduate and postgraduate courses in sport and exercise psychology and sport sociology. He is a registered sport psychologist and since 1998 has served as National Chair of the College of Sport Psychologists within the Australian Psychological Society. Over a 20-year period he has written and co-authored several book chapters and published papers that have assisted health professionals to both appreciate and apply a myriad of psychological factors associated with athletic injuries and, in particular, injury rehabilitation.

Peter Hamer is a Lecturer in Clinical Anatomy and Biomechanics in the Department of Human Movement and Exercise Science, The University of Western Australia, and is also the Director of the Functional Rehabilitation

Program (FRP), an exercise rehabilitation clinic within the same department. He has qualifications and practice experience in both physiotherapy and the exercise sciences and is currently completing his PhD in the above department investigating the mechanical, cellular, and tissue level responses that cause and/or prevent exercise-induced muscle damage.

Angela Hartman was a Johannson–Gund Research Scholar at the Mayo Clinic Sports Medicine Center, USA, at the time of publication, and is now pursuing her PhD in sport psychology at the University of Minnesota. She received her Master's degree from Western Illinois University, at which time she researched the influence of goal-setting in facilitating social support for injured athletes rehabilitating from injury. She has conducted applied sport psychology with a variety of both individual and team athletes and has worked in the clinical setting to enhance the coping skills of injured athletes.

Dr Gretchen A. Kerr is an Associate Professor and Associate Dean at the Faculty of Physical Education and Health, University of Toronto, Canada. Her research interests include the psychosocial aspects of athletic injury, both precipitating conditions and coping responses, particularly with respect to the experiences of young, competitive athletes. She teaches in the areas of psychosocial stress and child development and contributes to athlete and coach development through her work as a sport psychology consultant.

Dr Caroline Marlow is a Lecturer at the University of Surrey, UK, where she specializes in psychological techniques for the promotion of peak performance and motor control. Her PhD researched factors effecting adherence to psychological skills and fitness training in international cricketers. As a British Association of Sport and Exercise Science's (BASES) Accredited Sport Psychologist, Caroline works as a consultant to athletes from a variety of sports at a variety of levels. This includes the All England Netball Association and the University of Surrey, Roehampton's Sport Performance and Assessment Research Centre.

Dr Patricia Miller earned her doctorate in Exercise Science with a specialization in Sport Psychology at The University of Toronto, Canada. Her research interests focus on the psychosocial development of late adolescents through sport. She works as a sport psychology consultant in the university and local community with team and individual athletes and coaches.

Margaret Potter is a Lecturer in the School of Physiotherapy at Curtin University of Technology, Western Australia where she teaches communication skills and psychosocial issues relating to injury and rehabilitation to physiotherapy students. Also she works in private practice as a physiotherapist and injury rehabilitation consultant. She completed a MSc thesis examining the use of psychological skills during injury rehabilitation and is currently completing doctoral studies in the Department of Human Movement and Exercise Science at The University of Western Australia. The focus of her research is the difficult patient–physiotherapist interaction.

Dr Aynsley M. Smith is the sport psychology consultant and research director in the Mayo Clinic Sports Medicine Center, Rochester, Minnesota, USA. She is an Assistant Professor in the Departments of Orthopedic Surgery and Physical Medicine and Rehabilitation at the Mayo Medical School. Aynsley is an AAASP Certified Consultant and is on the AAASP Health Psychology Committee. She is an investigator on projects such as the relationship of psychophysiological factors to performance, the emotional response of athletes to injury, and on the epidemiology of injury. Aynsley has worked with hockey teams from Pee-Wee through professionals (NHL).

Dr Adrian Taylor is the Professor of Physical Activity and Health, School of Physical Education, Sport and Leisure at De Montfort University, UK. Since gaining a PhD in Exercise Science from the University of Toronto his main academic interests as a lecturer and researcher have focused on evaluating strategies to increase physical activity, psychological aspects of sports injury rehabilitation, and exercise and mental health. He has presented and published in academic and professional circles in North America, New Zealand, Israel, mainland Europe, and the UK on a variety of psychological topics related to leisure, sport, exercise, and health, over the past 18 years. He has been involved in training health professionals for many years. He is a BASES accredited psychologist.

Dr Eileen Udry is an Assistant Professor of Sport and Exercise Psychology at Indiana University Purdue University Indianapolis, Indiana, USA. Her work focuses on the psychology of athletic injuries. Specifically, she has conducted a number of research projects in collaboration with the US ski team and various sports medicine facilities. Additionally, she teaches a graduate class on the psychological aspects of sport injuries and rehabilitation and has consulted with elite and recreational athletes on the issue of injuries. Eileen's interests in injuries stems from her experience as a competitive, and now recreational athlete/exerciser.

Abbreviations

ACL	anterior cruciate ligament
AIMS	Athletic Identity Measurement Scale
AT	autogenic training
BFMP	body-fat measurement protocol
CT	computed tomography
EBP	evidence-based medicine/practice
EMG	electromyographic
ERAIQ	Emotional Response of Athletes to Injury Questionnaire
IER	intervention–evaluation review
MRI	magnetic resonance imaging
PMR	progressive muscular relaxation
POMR	Problem-oriented Medical Record
POMS	Profile of Mood States
QOL	quality of life
RAQ	Rehabilitation Adherence Questionnaire
RICE	rest, ice, compression, and elevation
RIPP	Rugby Injury and Performance Project (New Zealand)
SD	systematic desensitization
SICASS	Sports Injury Clinic, Athlete Satisfaction Scale
SIP	Sport Inventory for Pain
SIRBS	Sports Injury Rehabilitation Beliefs Survey
SIS	Sport Injury Survey
SIT	stress inoculation training
SMOC	The Sports Medicine Observation Code
SMP	sports medicine practitioners
SOAP	subjective–objective-assessment plan
TMD	total mood disturbance

*This book is dedicated to all injured athletes
who've ever asked themselves the question,
'Why me'?*

1 Emotional adjustment to sport injury

Britton W. Brewer

When athletes sustain injuries, the primary focus of sports medicine practitioners is, understandably, on the physical aspects of treatment and recovery. In addition to the physical consequences of sport injury, the psychological functioning of athletes may also be profoundly affected by injury. In particular, injury may have an impact on the emotional status of athletes. How athletes react emotionally to injury has important implications not only for their subjective well-being, but also for their rehabilitation behavior and clinical outcome.[1,2] Consequently, the purpose of this chapter is to present an overview of issues associated with the emotional adjustment of athletes to injury. Following a general description of emotional responses to sport injury, research on theoretical models of psychological response to sport injury, factors associated with emotional responses to sport injury, and potential consequences of emotional responses to sport injury are reviewed. Finally, strategies for recognizing poor emotional adjustment and facilitating positive emotional adjustment to sport injury are discussed.

Emotional responses to sport injury

Among the first to recognize the potentially devastating emotional impact of sport injury was Little,[3] who documented the disproportionate role of injury and illness as a precipitant of neurotic symptomatology in athletic males relative to non-athletic males. Little's seminal investigation set the stage for subsequent study of the emotional consequences of sport injury. Researchers have used both qualitative and quantitative methodologies to examine emotional responses to sport injury.

Qualitative findings

In qualitative studies of emotional aspects of sport injury, investigators ask injured athletes to recount their experiences over the course of rehabilitation. Through the use of qualitative methods, researchers have been able to obtain rich data on the emotional reactions incurred by athletes with injuries and the extent to which those emotions change during the rehabilitation process.

The period following sport injury has typically been described as one of emotional duress. Indeed, some athletes experiencing extreme depression after sustaining an injury have gone so far as to attempt suicide.[4] Across several studies, injured athletes have consistently described the early period of rehabilitation as marked by feelings of anger, confusion, depression, fear, and frustration.[5–9] Athletes have reported that as rehabilitation progresses, the negative emotions emanating most frequently from injury-related disruption of functioning tend to be depression and frustration. Reports of depression and frustration have been common even as rehabilitation nears completion and a return to sport is imminent. Athletes have cited the fear of reinjury as a salient emotion associated with resuming sport participation.[5,7] Thus, qualitative studies have documented a pattern of negative emotions in response to sport injury, with depression and frustration emerging as consistent themes throughout the rehabilitation process.

Quantitative findings

In quantitative studies of emotional responses to sport injury, researchers administer psychometric instruments (i.e. questionnaires) to athletes one or more times following injury and, in some cases, prior to injury as well. Quantitative data have been used to document emotional responses to sport injury, compare the responses of athletes with injuries to control samples (e.g. athletes without injuries), estimate the prevalence of clinically significant emotional disturbance following sport injury, and identify factors associated with emotional reactions to sport injury. The most frequently used measure of emotional status in quantitative investigations is the Profile of Mood States (POMS),[10] an instrument designed for use with general and clinical populations. Indices of emotional functioning specific to sport injury, such as the Emotional Responses of Athletes to Injury (ERAIQ)[11] and the Psychological Responses to Injury Inventory,[12] have also been developed for research use (see Chapter 2 for further information about assessment).

In general, the results of quantitative studies have indicated a tendency for negative emotions to decrease and positive emotions to increase over the course of rehabilitation.[13–24] However, two studies[15,25] have documented slight increases in negative emotions and slight decreases in positive emotions at the conclusion of a lengthy period of rehabilitation after knee surgery. Thus, although adverse emotional reactions tend to wane over time following injury, perhaps apprehension about resuming sport activity may trigger negative emotions as a return to sport participation approaches.

There are two lines of evidence from quantitative studies indicating that sport injury is associated with emotional disturbance. First, in studies comparing the emotional responses of injured and uninjured athletes, higher levels of emotional disturbance have been obtained for athletes with injuries.[16,19,26–34] Second, in investigations where preinjury and postinjury emotional functioning have been compared, greater emotional distress has been documented after the occurrence of injury.[16,19,34] Thus, although it cannot be definitively concluded that sport injury *causes* emotional disturbance, extant research findings suggest that such a relationship is highly likely.

By using standardized assessment instruments (e.g. the POMS) to measure emotional status, researchers have been able to estimate the extent to which athletes experience clinically meaningful emotional responses to injury. Results of epidemiological studies suggest that clinical levels of emotional disturbance are manifested by 5–24% of athletes with injuries.[16,26,31,35,36] The wide range of prevalence rates is probably a reflection of the different measures of emotional distress used and the samples examined. Nevertheless, it appears that although a sizable minority of postinjury emotional disturbance is of clinical proportions, most of the psychological distress experienced by injured athletes is subclinical in magnitude and duration. The subclinical nature of the bulk of postinjury emotional disturbance does not minimize its importance and adverse impact on athletes with injuries.

Perceptions of benefit associated with injury

Lest too negative a picture of emotional responses to injury be painted, it is important to note that not all athletes who sustain injuries experience negative emotional consequences and that some athletes even derive benefits in association with the occurrence and rehabilitation of their injuries.[37] Indeed, although injury can induce emotional turmoil, athletes have reported experiencing personal growth, challenge, and sport performance enhancement as a result of their injuries and subsequent rehabilitation.[9,38,39] For example, getting injured can heighten athletes' motivation for sport success and can provide them with opportunities to reflect, develop interests outside sport, test their character, and learn lessons about how their bodies work that can be put to use in training. Thus, experiencing injury can be potentially beneficial psychologically to some athletes.

Models of emotional response to sport injury

In an attempt to better understand how athletes react emotionally to injury, researchers have developed theoretical models of emotional response to sport injury. Theoretical models are used to guide both research and practice by directing attention to variables meriting study and to potential mechanisms of treatment success. Two general categories of theoretical models have emerged: stage models and cognitive appraisal models.

Stage models

Early writings on the psychological aspects of sport injury tended to endorse a stage-model approach to examining emotional and behavioral consequences of sport injury. Guided by the assumptions that injury can produce a loss of an aspect of the self and that athletes who sustain injuries experience a predictable sequence of psychological reactions, the model presented by Kubler-Ross[40] as a framework for understanding the psychological responses of persons with terminal illnesses was adapted to the realm of sport injury by several researchers.[41-43] In the adapted Kubler-Ross[40] model, athletes are proposed to proceed sequentially through stages of denial, anger, bargaining, and depression prior to accepting their injuries. The model has intuitive appeal, and has received empirical support to the extent that emotional responses to sport injury have been found to be compatible with those of a grief response[17] and that these are increasingly adaptive over the course of rehabilitation.[18,23]

The major problem with the adapted Kubler-Ross[40] model and other similar grief-based stage models is that they do not take into account individual differences in emotional reactions to sport injury. Research has failed to support the notion of a uniform, stage-like response not only to sport injury[1] but also to undesirable events in general.[44] Athletes experience a wide range of psychological reactions to injury. Assuming that an athlete is proceeding through a predictable series of stages following injury may be grossly inaccurate and potentially damaging to the patient–practitioner relationship. For example, athletes who do not appear to be emotionally distressed shortly after injury may, as the model suggests, be experiencing denial or, contrary to the model, may be adjusting quite well. Athletes who are erroneously treated as if they are in denial by their practitioners may become impatient or annoyed with their practitioners. Similarly, assuming that injured athletes 'should' encounter postinjury anger and depression may prompt medical practitioners to overlook potentially serious, negative emotional reactions to injury as 'normal' or 'expected' and consequently fail to address the athletes' psychological concerns. Although some proponents of stage models have specified that individuals can move back and forth through the various stages,[45] such specifications limit the predictive utility of stage models[46] unless the conditions under which movements occur across stages are identified. In other words, there is little benefit to the concept of stages if it cannot be specified what causes individuals to be in a particular stage and what will prompt them to change to a different stage.

Cognitive appraisal models

Recognizing the limitations of stage models in accounting for individual differences in psychological reactions to sport injury, a number of researchers have used cognitive appraisal models, which originated in the literature on stress and coping, to guide their work on emotional responses to sport injury.[1,2] As depicted in Fig. 1.1, the central tenet of cognitive appraisal models as applied to sport injury is that emotional and behavioral responses

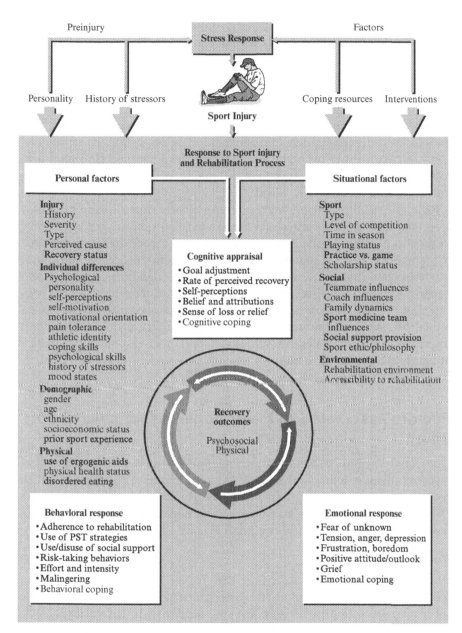

Fig. 1.1 Integrated model of psychological response to the sport injury and rehabilitation process. (Reprinted with permission from Wiese-Bjornstal, D. M., Smith, A. M., Shaffer, S. M., and Morrey, M. A. (1998). An integrated model of response to sport injury: psychological and sociological dimensions. *Journal of Applied Sport Psychology*, **10**, 46–69. Copyright 1998 by the Association for the Advancement of Applied Sport Psychology.)

to sport injury influence and, more importantly, are influenced by cognitive interpretations (or appraisals) of the injury situation. Thus, whether athletes perceive their injuries as threats or as challenges may have a profound impact on how they feel and act during rehabilitation. Further, as shown in Fig. 1.1, cognitive appraisals are thought to be influenced by characteristics of the injured individual and the situational context in which injury rehabilitation occurs. It is important to note that cognitive appraisal models are dynamic and, as such, the magnitude and direction of relations among key model components may vary over time. For example, the potential influence of pain tolerance on postinjury depression may diminish as rehabilitation progresses and acute pain becomes less salient.

Research findings have provided general support for predictions generated from cognitive appraisal models.[1,2] For the most part, however, the evidence in support of these models has been correlational rather than experimental. More rigorous tests of cognitive appraisal models are needed before causal inferences can be made about the relations among cognitions, emotions, and behaviors in sport injury rehabilitation. Nevertheless, these models offer considerable promise as a means of explaining psychological responses to sport injury. Moreover, consistent with clinical and empirical observations that injured athletes sometimes exhibit elements of a grief response,[17] cognitive appraisal models can be used to understand why such reactions might occur without the 'baggage' associated with stage models.[2,47]

Factors associated with emotional responses to sport injury

One important implication of cognitive appraisal models of psychological response to sport injury is that there are a multitude of factors thought to contribute to postinjury emotional reactions. Research has substantiated this claim. In particular, numerous personal, situational, and cognitive variables have been linked to emotional responses to sport injury in scientific studies.

Personal factors

Personal factors are characteristics that remain fairly stable over time. Athletes who experience emotional disturbance following injury tend to be those who are young,[23,35,48] who strongly identify with the athlete role,[8,49] invest in playing professional sport,[50] are competitive (versus recreational) athletes,[48] less hardy,[19] and knowledgeable about or experienced in the physical consequences of the injury.[5]

Situational factors

Unlike personal factors, situational factors typically vary extensively over time. Some of the situational variables that have been associated with emotional disturbance following sport injury pertain to the characteristics of the injury itself. Athletes are more likely to experience postinjury emotional distress when their injuries are acute,[35,51] severe,[5,7,23,24,34,52] uncommon,[5] and less fully healed.[7,18,51,53] Other situational variables that have been linked to affective responses to sport injury have to do with the circumstances in which the injury occurred. Athletes have tended to report greater emotional disturbance when they are participating at a low level of competition[13] and who sustain their injuries at a particularly inopportune time of the season.[5] Emotional disturbance is also more likely to occur in conjunction with sport injury when the athletes perceive their injuries as impairing their daily activities,[54] and perceive themselves under a high degree of life stress[49,51] and lacking social support.[49,51,55]

Cognitive factors

Consistent with a cognitive appraisal view of psychological responses to sport injury, a variety of cognitive variables have been associated with emotional reactions to sport injury. In particular, emotional disturbance has been more common among athletes who perceive themselves as having difficulty coping with their injuries,[56] have a low regard for themselves[51] and their physical abilities,[49] lack confidence in themselves and their ability to adhere to their rehabilitation program, be successful at sport, and recover fully from their injuries.[51] Also, athletes who attributed the cause of their injuries to internal factors tended to report higher levels of emotional disturbance in one study[57] and lower levels of emotional disturbance in another.[58] Thus, it is unclear whether self-blame for injury is adaptive or maladaptive in emotional responses to sport injury.

Results of a recent study[7] suggest that cognitive appraisals have important implications for emotional functioning throughout the sport injury rehabilitation process. Appraisals of injury severity, treatment efficacy, rehabilitation progress, risk of returning to sport, and missed opportunities and goals due to injury were found to be closely linked with postinjury emotions. Both the valence and type of cognitive appraisals were related to specific emotional responses. For example, whereas negative appraisals of rehabilitation progress were associated with apathy, depression, and frustration, positive appraisals were associated with happiness and relief. Conversely, negative appraisals of treatment efficacy (i.e. beliefs that the rehabilitation regimen was not working) were commonly accompanied by dissatisfaction and anger.

As proposed in cognitive appraisal models, cognitive responses to injury are thought to mediate the relationship between emotional responses and various personal and situational factors. That is, personal and situational factors are presumed to influence emotions not so much directly as indirectly by affecting how athletes think about their injuries and themselves in relation to their injuries. Research has provided support for this hypothesis, indicating that postinjury cognitions have been associated with a host of personal and situational variables. Illustrating the relationship between personal and cognitive factors, significant correlations have been documented between:

(1) psychological investment in playing sport professionally and postinjury self-esteem (a self-referent cognition);[50]

(2) having experienced previous successful rehabilitation in the past and rehabilitation self-efficacy;[59]

(3) neuroticism (a personality characteristic) and selected cognitive coping strategies.[60]

Situational factors have also been linked to postinjury cognitions. In particular, significant relationships have been reported between:

(1) daily hassles (an indicator of life stress) and self-confidence;[22]

(2) social support and self-confidence;[22]

(3) stage of rehabilitation and self-confidence;[22] and

(4) stage of rehabilitation and emotion-focused coping strategies.[61]

Summary

Qualitative and quantitative research methods have been used to document the wide variety of personal, situational, and cognitive factors associated with the emotional state of athletes following injury. Because the data providing support for the obtained relationships are without exception correlational in nature, inferences cannot be made regarding the causal role of personal characteristics, the situational context in which injury rehabilitation occurs, and cognitive appraisals in producing postinjury emotional distress. Nevertheless, medical practitioners can apply knowledge of those factors most likely to be related to poor emotional adjustment to identify warning signs in athletes who are at risk for a postinjury affective disturbance.

Potential consequences of emotional responses to sport injury

Almost by definition, negative emotional reactions to sport injury are aversive experiences in and of themselves. When athletes encounter anger, depression, or frustration upon becoming injured, the emotional response has important implications for both their psychological and physical functioning. From a cognitive appraisal perspective, emotional responses to injury are thought to influence behavioral responses to injury and rehabilitation outcomes.

Emotional responses and adherence to sport injury rehabilitation programs

The behavioral response to sport injury that has been examined most extensively is adherence to rehabilitation, which involves engaging in behaviors such as restricting physical activity, completing home exercises, complying with medication prescriptions, and participating in clinic-based rehabilitation exercises and therapy.[62,63] Adherence can be an important contributor to the outcome of such rehabilitation programs.[51,64–67] In two studies, emotional disturbance was inversely related to sport injury rehabilitation adherence,[56,68] suggesting that negative emotions may interfere with the ability of athletes to complete the tasks assigned to them by medical practitioners.

Emotional responses and sport injury rehabilitation outcomes

Negative emotions may exert an adverse influence not only on rehabilitation behaviors but also on rehabilitation outcomes. Although cognitive appraisal models such as that depicted in Fig. 1.1 show proposed relationships between specific psychological factors, they generally do not offer explanations for how psychological factors, such as emotions, affect sport injury rehabilitation outcomes. In contrast, the biopsychosocial model of sport injury rehabilitation[69] displayed in Fig. 1.2 offers a broad-based framework for understanding the potential contribution of emotional reactions to physical recovery from sport injury. This model proposes that psychological factors, including emotional responses to sport injury, affect rehabilitation outcomes both directly and indirectly through their interactions with biological factors and intermediate biopsychological outcomes (e.g. range of motion, strength, joint laxity, pain, endurance, recovery rate). In support of this hypothesis, research has documented significant relationships between emotional variables and sport injury rehabilitation outcomes. Higher levels of general well-being[70,71] and vigor[51] have been associated with more favorable rehabilitation outcomes. Conversely, higher levels of injury rehabilitation anxiety,[70,71] psychological distress,[64] anger, fear, and frustration[15] have been associated with less favorable rehabilitation outcomes.

Thus, it appears that positive and negative emotions have an opposite pattern of relations with recovery from sport injury. As with research on predictors of emotional responses to sport injury, the findings for the relationship between emotional factors and rehabilitation outcomes are correlational and preclude causal inferences from being drawn. Nevertheless, the pattern of results is wholly consistent with that predicted by the biopsychosocial model.[69]

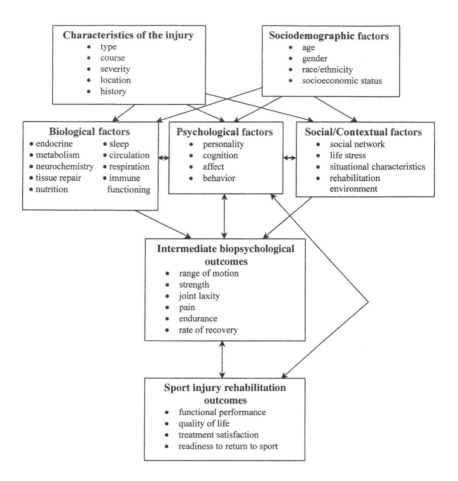

Fig. 1.2 A biopsychosocial model of sport injury rehabilitation. (Reproduced with permission from Brewer, B. W., Andersen, M. B., and Van Raalte, J. L. Psychological aspects of sport injury rehabilitation: toward a biopsychosocial approach. In *Medical aspects of sport and exercise* (ed. D. I. Mostofsky and L. D. Zaichkowsky). Fitness Information Technology, Morgantown, WV. (In press.)

Interventions to facilitate positive emotional adjustment to sport injury

Petitpas and Danish[72] identified 14 psychological interventions that have been suggested to help athletes adjust to injury, including biofeedback, goal-setting, imagery, progressive relaxation, psychotherapy, and systematic desensitization (see Chapters 6 and 7 for further information). From a cognitive appraisal perspective,[1,2,47] the interventions are thought to influence postinjury emotions by altering cognitions and behaviors that bear directly on emotional functioning. Although empirical research on the efficacy of these interventions is limited, the few investigations that have been conducted have provided data supporting the use of psychological treatments in sport injury rehabilitation.[73]

It is important to note that the appropriate individual to implement a psychological intervention depends greatly on the psychological state of the injured athlete and the nature of the intervention. For athletes experiencing mild postinjury dysphoria, a straightforward intervention—such as electromyographic (EMG) biofeedback, goal-setting, imagery, positive self-talk, or progressive relaxation might be implemented by a medical practitioner (with specialized sport psychology training). This may help athletes reduce their distress by decreasing their sense of helplessness and focusing them more clearly on the tasks of the rehabilitation regimen. For athletes with more severe emotional adjustment difficulties who may require more extensive psychological treatment (e.g., counseling, psychotherapy), a mental health professional would be the appropriate individual to initiate the psychological intervention.

Recognition and referral of athletes with poor emotional adjustment to sport injury

Because of the adverse impact that pronounced and prolonged negative emotional states can have on psychological and physical functioning, it is important for those having the most contact with injured athletes to be able to identify poor emotional adjustment to sport injury and make referrals for psychological treatment when necessary. Given their proximity to these athletes throughout the rehabilitation process, medical practitioners are well positioned to recognize athletes who experience emotional adjustment difficulties after sustaining an injury. Despite their regular contact with athletes undergoing injury rehabilitation, medical practitioners may believe they lack sufficient knowledge to determine when athletes are experiencing emotional disturbance and thus feel uncomfortable about even discussing the issue with athletes, much less making a referral for psychological services. Supporting this position are the results of a study in which medical practitioners' observations of patients' postinjury psychological distress were not significantly correlated with patients' ratings of their own postinjury psychological distress.[36] It is unclear whether the lack of agreement between the practitioners' observations and the patients' ratings was due to the patients' concealment of their distress from the practitioners, the practitioners' lack of confidence in their ability to make judgments about the psychological state of their patients, the measures of psychological distress that were used, or some combination of these and other factors. Nevertheless, there is undoubtedly value to having medical practitioners feel confident and competent in evaluating the possibility that certain athletes under their care may need some sort of psychological assistance to enhance their emotional adjustment to injury and, ultimately, their treatment outcome.

Although there is a small but consistent percentage of athletes who encounter difficulty adjusting emotionally to injury,[16,26,31,35,36] their referral by medical practitioners to mental health services is far from routine. A study of sports medicine physicians revealed that most had referred at least one of their patients for psychological evaluation or treatment.[74] In contrast, the majority of athletic trainers surveyed in a recent study had never referred an athlete for psychological services, and had no standard procedures for doing so should the need arise.[75] Thus, professionals, who in many cases have day-to-day contact with athletes undergoing injury rehabilitation, may be unprepared to make appropriate psychological referrals. Although formal training in the psychological aspects of sport injury has been proposed as a standard part of the education of medical practitioners,[76] such training is not yet widespread.

Guidelines for the recognition and referral of athletes experiencing difficulty adjusting emotionally to injury have been offered by several authors.[78-80] In some instances, recognizing emotional adjustment difficulties may be as simple as noticing when injured athletes display overt signs of significant emotional distress such as depression, anger, and frustration. However, because athletes can often keep their emotions under control in the rehabilitation environment, identification of emotional disturbances may require making inferences from athletes' rehabilitation behavior (e.g. adhering poorly to the rehabilitation program, denying the seriousness of an injury, overdoing rehabilitation), and reports (from the athletes themselves or from others) of behaviors and occurrences outside the rehabilitation context (e.g. impaired functioning in important life domains, sleep disturbance).[72,80] Medical practitioners can obtain information beyond the typical physical focus of rehabilitation by asking athletes informally about how they are dealing with their injuries, how they are sleeping, how things are going in other areas of their lives (e.g. school, work, social relationships), how they feel about their rehabilitation progress, and other pertinent matters. Of course, such inquiry can be greatly facilitated by first establishing rapport with and gaining the trust of athletes with injuries.[72]

Once those athletes who could potentially benefit from referral for psychological services have been identified, it can be useful for medical professionals to consult with a mental health practitioner (who may or may not have an affiliation with the sports medicine team) for guidance on an appropriate course of action. The mental health practitioner may suggest that the medical practitioner gather additional information, carry out a trial intervention (e.g. teaching progressive muscle relaxation skills), or make an immediate referral.

If a referral is suggested, the timing of the referral is likely to be influenced by such factors as the severity of the athlete's symptoms, the athlete's coping resources, the medical practitioner's skills and training, the relationship between the medical practitioner and the athlete, the relationship between the medical practitioner and the mental health professional, and other characteristics of the rehabilitation environment (e.g. privacy) and situation (e.g. athlete's current emotional state).[77] Optimally, prior to referral, medical practitioners will have established a relationship with a mental health professional who is skilled in treating emotional adjustment difficulties in athletes and in whom they are confident. Because referral for psychological services can be a sensitive process, it is vital for medical practitioners to be aware of athletes' potential concerns about the relevance of referral to their rehabilitation and about being stigmatized for consulting a mental health professional. Athletes receiving referrals can be reassured that they are not being viewed as 'head cases' and that addressing psychological issues can facilitate the successful physical rehabilitation of sport injuries.[79] When athletes refuse a referral, it is appropriate to again suggest the possibility of referral at a later time when they may be more receptive to the idea.

Once athletes who have difficulty in adjusting emotionally to their injury have been referred to a mental health professional, medical practitioners can follow up the athletes about their treatment and, with the athletes' consent, discuss their progress in general terms with their rehabilitation professional.[77] Such follow-up enables the medical practitioners to coordinate the care of the athletes to best meet their physical and psychological needs.

Summary and conclusions

Sport injury can have a profound impact on the emotional functioning of athletes. Emotional disturbance, predominantly of a subclinical nature, following sport injury is not uncommon. Typical negative emotional reactions to injury include elevations in anger, depression, and frustration. How athletes respond emotionally to injury is influenced by their personal characteristics, the situations in which the injury and injury rehabilitation occur, and, perhaps most importantly, the cognitive interpretations the athletes attach to their injuries.

Because emotional responses to sport injury are highly variable both across individuals and over time, it should not be automatically assumed that athletes with injuries are experiencing emotional disturbance. Doing so normalizes postinjury psychological distress and may cause significant emotional disturbance to go unaddressed. Conversely, because it is not unusual for athletes to experience negative emotions following injury, it is essential to avoid labeling mild or transient dysphoria as a disorder—while being on the lookout for emotional adjustment difficulties warranting clinical attention.

Problems adjusting emotionally to sport injury can hamper athletes' adherence to and physical outcomes gained from rehabilitation programs. Psychological interventions, some of which can be implemented by medical practitioners and some of which require referral to a mental health professional, can ameliorate the effects of adverse emotional reactions to sport injury. Because negative mood states are a risk factor for incurring a sport injury,[81] interventions targeted at reducing emotional disturbance during injury rehabilitation can be viewed as preventive with respect to reinjury. Referrals to mental health professionals for psychological services, when needed, should be handled with care.[77–80]

To ignore the emotional impact of sport injury is to neglect an important facet of the subjective experience of rehabilitation. By attending to the emotional responses of athletes to injury, more comprehensive treatment is likely to result and the athletes are likely to be better served both physically and psychologically.

Acknowledgment

Preparation of this chapter was supported in part by grant number R29 AR44484 from the National Institute of Arthritis and Musculoskeletal and Skin Diseases. Its contents are solely the responsibility of the author and do not represent the official views of the National Institute of Arthritis and Musculoskeletal and Skin Diseases.

References

1. Brewer, B. W. (1994). Review and critique of models of psychological adjustment to athletic injury. *Journal of Applied Sport Psychology*, **6**, 87–100.
2. Wiese-Bjornstal, D. M., Smith, A. M., Shaffer, S. M., and Morrey, M. A. (1998). An integrated model of response to sport injury: Psychological and sociological dimensions. *Journal of Applied Sport Psychology*, **10**, 46–69.
3. Little, J. C. (1969). The athlete's neurosis—a deprivation crisis. *Acta Psychiatrica Scandinavia*, **45**, 187–97.
4. Smith, A. M. and Milliner, E. K. (1994). Injured athletes and the risk of suicide. *Journal of Athletic Training*, **29**, 337–41.
5. Bianco, T., Malo, S., and Orlick, T. (1999). Sport injury and illness: Elite skiers describe their experiences. *Research Quarterly for Exercise and Sport*, **70**, 157–69.
6. Gordon, S. and Lindgren, S. (1990). Psycho-physical rehabilitation from a serious sport injury: Case study of an elite fast bowler. *Australian Journal of Science and Medicine in Sport*, **22**, 71–6.
7. Johnston, L. H. and Carroll, D. (1998). The context of emotional responses to athletic injury: A qualitative analysis. *Journal of Sport Rehabilitation*, **7**, 206–20.

8. Sparkes, A. C. (1998). An Achilles heel to the survival of self. *Qualitative Health Research*, **8**, 644–64.
9. Udry, E., Gould, D., Bridges, D., and Beck, L. (1997). Down but not out: Athlete responses to season-ending injuries. *Journal of Sport* and *Exercise Psychology*, **19**, 229–48.
10. McNair, D. M., Lorr, M., and Droppleman, L. F. (1971). *Manual for the profile of mood states.* Educational and Industrial Testing Service, San Diego, CA.
11. Smith, A. M., Scott, S. G., and Wiese, D. M. (1990). The psychological effects of sports injuries. Coping. *Sports Medicine*, **9**, 352–69.
12. Evans, L., Hardy, L., and Mullen, R. (1996). The development of the psychological responses to injury inventory. *Journal of Sports Sciences*, **14**, 27–8. [Abstract]
13. Crossman, J., Gluck, L., and Jamieson, J. (1995) The emotional responses of injured athletes. *New Zealand Journal of Sports Medicine*, **23**, 1–2.
14. Dawes, H. and Roach, N. K. (1997). Emotional responses of athletes to injury and treatment. *Physiotherapy*, **83**, 243–7.
15. LaMott, E. E. (1994). *The anterior cruciate ligament injured athlete: the psychological process.* PhD thesis, University of Minnesota, Minneapolis.
16. Leddy, M. H., Lambert, M. J., and Ogles, B. M. (1994). Psychological consequences of athletic injury among high-level competitors. *Research Quarterly for Exercise and Sport*, **65**, 347–54.
17. Macchi, R. and Crossman, J. (1996). After the fall: Reflections of injured classical ballet dancers. *Journal of Sport Behaviour*, **19**, 221–34.
18. McDonald, S. A. and Hardy, C. J. (1990). Affective response patterns of the injured athlete: An exploratory analysis. *The Sport Psychologist*, **4**, 261–74.
19. Miller, W. N. (1998). Athletic injury: mood disturbances and hardiness of intercollegiate athletes. *Journal of Applied Sport Psychology*, **10**(Suppl.), S127–8. [Abstract]
20. Morrey, M. A. (1997). *A longitudinal examination of emotional response, cognitive coping, and physical recovery among athletes undergoing anterior cruciate ligament reconstructive surgery.* PhD thesis, University of Minnesota, Minneapolis.
21. Quackenbush, N. and Crossman, J. (1994). Injured athletes: A study of emotional response. *Journal of Sport Behavior*, **17**, 178–87.
22. Quinn, A. M. and Fallon, B. J. (1999). The changes in psychological characteristics and reactions of elite athletes from injury onset until full recovery. *Journal of Applied Sport Psychology*, **11**, 210–29.
23. Smith, A. M., Scott, S. G., O'Fallon, W. M., and Young, M. L. (1990). Emotional responses of athletes to injury. *Mayo Clinic Proceedings*, **65**, 38–50.
24. Uemukai, K. (1993). Affective responses and the changes in athletes due to injury. In *Proceedings of the 8th World Congress of Sport Psychology* (ed. S. Serpa, J. Alves, V. Ferreira, and A. Paula-Brito), pp. 500–3. International Society of Sport Psychology, Lisbon, Portugal.

25. Morrey, M. A., Stuart, M. J., Smith, A. M., and Wiese-Bjornstal, D. M. (1999). A longitudinal examination of athletes' emotional and cognitive responses to anterior cruciate ligament injury. *Clinical Journal of Sport Medicine*, **9**, 63–9.

26. Brewer, B. W. and Petrie, T. A. (1995). A comparison between injured and uninjured football players on selected psychosocial variables. *Academic Athletic Journal*, **10**, 11–18.

27. Chan, C. S. and Grossman, H. Y. (1988). Psychological effects of running loss on consistent runners. *Perceptual and Motor Skills*, **66**, 875–83.

28. Johnson, U. (1998). Psychological risk factors during the rehabilitation of competitive male soccer players with serious knee injuries. *Journal of Sports Sciences*, **16**, 391–2. [Abstract]

29. Johnson, U. (1997) Coping strategies among long-term injured competitive athletes. A study of 81 men and women in team and individual sports. *Scandinavian Journal of Medicine* and *Science in Sports, 7*, 367–372.

30. Pearson, L. and Jones, G. (1992). Emotional effects of sports injuries: Implications for physiotherapists. *Physiotherapy*, **78**, 762–70.

31. Perna, F. M., Roh, J., Newcomer, R. R., and Etzel, E. F. (1998). Clinical depression among injured athletes: An empirical assessment. *Journal of Applied Sport Psychology*, **10**(Suppl.), S54–5. [Abstract]

32. Petrie, T. A., Brewer, B., and Buntrock, C. (1997). A comparison between injured and uninjured NCAA Division I male and female athletes on selected psychosocial variables. *Journal of Applied Sport Psychology*, **9**(Suppl.), S144. [Abstract]

33. Roh, J., Newcomer, R. R., Perna, F. M., and Etzel, E. F. (1998). Depressive mood states among college athletes: Pre- and post-injury. *Journal of Applied Sport Psychology*, **10**(Suppl.), S54. [Abstract]

34. Smith, A. M., Stuart, M. J., Wiese-Bjornstal, D. M., Milliner, E. K., O'Fallon, W. M., and Crowson, C. S. (1993). Competitive athletes: Preinjury and postinjury mood state and self-esteem. *Mayo Clinic Proceedings*, **68**, 939–47.

35. Brewer, B. W., Linder, D. E., and Phelps, C. M. (1995). Situational correlates of emotional adjustment to athletic injury. *Clinical Journal of Sport Medicine*, **5**, 241–5.

36. Brewer, B. W., Petitpas, A. J., Van Raalte, J. L., Sklar, J. H., and Ditmar, T. D. (1995). Prevalence of psychological distress among patients at a physical therapy clinic specializing in sports medicine. *Sports Medicine, Training and Rehabilitation*, **6**, 138–45.

37. Udry, E. (1999). The paradox of injuries: Unexpected positive consequences. In *Psychological bases of sport injuries* (2nd edn) (ed. D. Pargman), pp. 79–88. Fitness Information Technology, Morgantown, WV.

38. Ford, I. W. and Gordon, S. (1999). Coping with sport injury: Resource loss and the role of social support. *Journal of Personal and Interpersonal Loss*, **4**, 243–56.

39. Rose, J. and Jevne, R. F. J. (1993). Psychosocial processes associated with sport injuries. *The Sport Psychologist*, **7**, 309–28.

40. Kubler-Ross, E. (1969). *On death and dying.* Macmillan, New York.
41. Astle, S. J. (1986). The experience of loss in athletes. *Journal of Sports Medicine and Physical Fitness*, **26**, 279–84.
42. Lynch, G. P. (1988). Athletic injuries and the practicing sport psychologist: Practical guidelines for assisting athletes. *The Sport Psychologist*, **2**, 161–7.
43. Rotella, B. (1985). The psychological care of the injured athlete. In *Sport psychology: psychological considerations in maximizing sport performance* (ed. L. K. Bunker, R. J. Rotella, and A. S. Reilly), pp. 273–87. Mouvement, Ann Arbor, MI.
44. Silver, R. L. and Wortman, C. B. (1980). Coping with undesirable events. In *Human helplessness: theory and applications* (ed. J. Garber and M. E. P. Seligman), pp. 279–375. Academic Press, New York.
45. Evans, L. and Hardy, L. (1995). Sport injury and grief responses: A review. *Journal of Sport* and *Exercise Psychology*, **17**, 227–45.
46. Rape, R. N., Bush, J. P., and Slavin, L. A. (1992). Toward a conceptualization of the family's adaptation to a member's head injury: a critique of developmental stage models. *Rehabilitation Psychology*, **37**, 3–22.
47. Evans, L. and Hardy, L. (1999). Psychological and emotional response to athletic injury: Measurement issues. In *Psychological bases of sport injuries* (2nd edn) (ed. D. Pargman), pp. 49–64. Fitness Information Technology, Morgantown, WV.
48. Meyers, M. C., Sterling, J. C., Calvo, R. D., Marley, R., and Duhon, T. K. (1991). Mood state of athletes undergoing orthopaedic surgery and rehabilitation: A preliminary report. *Medicine and Science in Sports and Exercise*, **23**(Suppl.), S138.
49. Brewer, B. W. (1993). Self-identity and specific vulnerability to depressed mood. *Journal of Personality*, **61**, 343–64.
50. Kleiber, D. A. and Brock, S. C. (1992). The effect of career-ending injuries on the subsequent well-being of elite college athletes. *Sociology of Sport Journal*, **9**, 70–5.
51. Quinn, A. M. (1996). *The psychological factors involved in the recovery of elite athletes from long term injuries.* PhD thesis, University of Melbourne, Australia.
52. Pargman, D. and Lunt, S. D. (1989). The relationship of self-concept and locus of control to the severity of injury in freshmen collegiate football players. *Sports Training, Medicine and Rehabilitation*, **1**, 203–8.
53. Smith, A. M., Young, M. L., and Scott, S. G. (1988). The emotional responses of athletes to injury. *Canadian Journal of Sport Sciences*, **13**(Suppl.), 84P–5P.
54. Crossman, J. and Jamieson, J. (1985). Differences in perceptions of seriousness and disrupting effects of athletic injury as viewed by athletes and their trainer. *Perceptual and Motor Skills*, **61**, 1131–4.
55. Green, S. L. and Weinberg, R. S. (1998). The relationship between athletic identity, coping skills, social support, and the psychological impact of injury. *Journal of Applied Sport Psychology*, **10**(Suppl.), S127. [Abstract]

56. Daly, J. M., Brewer, B. W., Van Raalte, J. L., Petitpas, A. J., and Sklar, J. H. (1995). Cognitive appraisal, emotional adjustment, and adherence to rehabilitation following knee surgery. *Journal of Sport Rehabilitation*, **4**, 23–30.

57. Tedder, S. and Biddle, S. J. H. (1998). Psychological processes involved during sports injury rehabilitation: An attribution–emotion investigation. *Journal of Sports Sciences*, **16**, 106–7. [Abstract]

58. Brewer, B. W. (1999). Causal attribution dimensions and adjustment to sport injury. *Journal of Personal and Interpersonal Loss*, **4**, 215–24.

59. Shaffer, S. M. (1992). *Attributions and self-efficacy as predictors of rehabilitative success*. Master's thesis, University of Illinois, Champaign.

60. Grove, J. R., Bahnsen, A., and Eklund, R. C. (1997). Neuroticism, injury severity, and coping with rehabilitation. In *Innovations in sport psychology: linking theory and practice* (Part I) (ed. R. Lidor and M. Bar-Eli), pp. 298–300. International Society of Sport Psychology, Netanya, Israel.

61. Udry, E. (1997). Coping and social support among injured athletes following surgery. *Journal of Sport* and *Exercise Psychology*, **19**, 71–90.

62. Brewer, B. W. (1998). Adherence to sport injury rehabilitation programs. *Journal of Applied Sport Psychology*, **10**, 70–82.

63. Brewer, B. W. (1999). Adherence to sport injury rehabilitation regimens. In *Adherence issues in sport and exercise* (ed. S. J. Bull), pp. 145–68). Wiley, Chichester.

64. Brewer, B. W., Van Raalte, J. L., Cornelius, A. E., Petitpas, A. J., Sklar, J. H., Pohlman, M. H., Krushell, R. J., and Ditmar, T. D. (2000). Psychological factors, rehabilitation adherence, and rehabilitation outcome following anterior cruciate ligament reconstruction. *Rehabilitation Psychology*, **45**, 20–37.

65. Derscheid, G. L. and Feiring, D. C. (1987). A statistical analysis to characterize treatment adherence of the 18 most common diagnoses seen at a sports medicine clinic. *Journal of Orthopaedic and Sports Physical Therapy*, **9**, 40–6.

66. Treacy, S. H., Barron, O. A., Brunet, M. E., and Barrack, R. L. (1997). Assessing the need for extensive supervised rehabilitation following arthroscopic surgery. *American Journal of Orthopedics*, **26**, 25–9.

67. Tuffey, S. (1991). *The use of psychological skills to facilitate recovery from athletic injury*. Master's thesis, University of North Carolina, Greensboro.

68. Brickner, J. C. (1997). *Mood states and compliance of patients with orthopedic rehabilitation*. Master's thesis, Springfield College, MA.

69. Brewer, B. W., Andersen, M. B., and Van Raalte, J. L. Psychological aspects of sport injury rehabilitation: Toward a biopsychosocial approach. In *Medical aspects of sport and exercise* (ed. D. I. Mostofsky and L. D. Zaichkowsky). Fitness Information Technology, Morgantown, WV. (In press.)

70. Johnson, U. (1996). Quality of experience of long-term injury in athletic sports predicts return after rehabilitation. In *Aktuell beteendevetenskaplig idrottsforskning* (ed. G. Patriksson), pp. 110–17. SVEBI, Lund, Sweden.

71. Johnson, U. (1997). A three-year follow-up of long-term injured competitive

athletes: Influence of psychological risk factors on rehabilitation. *Journal of Sport Rehabilitation*, **6**, 256–71.

72. Petitpas, A. and Danish, S. J. (1995). Caring for injured athletes. In *Sport psychology interventions* (ed. S. M. Murphy), pp. 255–81. Human Kinetics, Champaign, IL.
73. Cupal, D. D. (1998). Psychological interventions in sport injury prevention and rehabilitation. *Journal of Applied Sport Psychology*, **10**, 103–23.
74. Brewer, B. W., Van Raalte, J. L., and Linder, D. E. (1991). Role of the sport psychologist in treating injured athletes: A survey of sports medicine providers. *Journal of Applied Sport Psychology*, **3**, 183–90.
75. Larson, G. A., Starkey, C. A., and Zaichkowsky, L. D. (1996). Psychological aspects of athletic injuries as perceived by athletic trainers. *The Sport Psychologist*, **10**, 37–47.
76. Gordon, S., Potter, M., and Ford, I. (1998). Toward a psychoeducational curriculum for training sport-injury rehabilitation personnel. *Journal of Applied Sport Psychology*, **10**, 140–56.
77. Brewer, B. W., Petitpas, A. J., and Van Raalte, J. L. (1999). Referral of injured athletes for counseling and psychotherapy. In *Counseling in sports medicine* (ed. R. Ray and D. M. Wiese-Bjornstal), pp. 127–41. Human Kinetics, Champaign, IL.
78. Brewer, B. W., Van Raalte, J. L., and Petitpas, A. J. (1999). Patient–practitioner interactions in sport injury rehabilitation. In *Psychological bases of sport injuries* (2nd edn) (ed. D. Pargman), pp. 157–74. Fitness Information Technology, Morgantown, WV.
79. Heil, J. (1993). Referral and coordination of care. In *Psychology of sport injury* (ed. J. Heil), pp. 251–66. Human Kinetics, Champaign, IL.
80. Taylor, J. and Taylor, S. (1997). *Psychological approaches to sports injury rehabilitation.* Aspen, Gaithersburg, MD.
81. Williams, J. M. and Andersen, M. B. (1998). Psychosocial antecedents of sport injury: Review and critique of the stress and injury model. *Journal of Applied Sport Psychology*, **10**, 5–25.

2 *Assessment of the injured athlete*

Aynsley M. Smith, Angela D. Hartman, and Nicole J. Detling

Introduction

The number of reported athletic injuries has increased[1,2] as a consequence of more people becoming involved in sports and improved methods of detecting and diagnosing injuries. The fact that athletes are participating in sports at younger ages, thus identifying themselves as athletes early in life, makes both acute and chronic injury more devastating. Frequently, athletes of all ages have their dreams and goals interrupted by injury. When injuries are severe,[3,4] athletes may have legitimate doubts about whether they will be able to return to their preinjury level of performance.[5,6]

Although many athletic injuries are very serious, the physical and psychological repercussions of catastrophic injuries (defined as an event, either sports or non-sports related, that brings about a sudden and permanent end to sport participation) are the most damaging.[7] When a catastrophic injury occurs, the injured athlete may immediately realize that sport participation as an able-bodied person is no longer possible. For example, during the winter of 1999, a ski instructor was teaching a speed class at a downhill ski resort. This accomplished 28-year-old instructor lost an edge at high speed, slid down a headwall, and crashed into a cedar post at the bottom of the run. When the ski patrol arrived on the scene, the skier had no sensation in his lower body. He lost consciousness and did not recall his emergency transportation to the hospital. Upon regaining consciousness that evening, he gradually became aware that the worst fears of an athletically identified,[8] high-energy, competent, thrill-seeking, young man had been realized. He was paralyzed from the waist down.

As a result of the various levels of frustration, depression, and anger commonly associated with injury,[3,5,9–15] it is important to assess the psychosocial response of the athletes, particularly those with serious injuries.[16] Often, when mood disturbance (accounted for by high depression, tension, anger, fatigue, and low vigor) is severe,[4] so much energy is spent trying to re-establish emotional equilibrium (psychological) that little energy is available for rehabilitation (physical).

The goal of the assessment interview[16] is to gain an understanding of the athlete's perception of his or her injury,[17] emotional response, social support system,[18] and sources of stress,[19,20] as well as the factors affecting the athlete's ability to cope with the injury[21] and subsequent rehabilitation and recovery process.[5,22–32]

A rationale for an integrated psychosocial and physical assessment

The purpose of this chapter is to provide a rationale for the assessment of the injured athlete. Although this chapter focuses primarily on assessment of the psychosocial aspects of injury, it assumes that the medical practitioner (physician, physical therapist, athletic trainer, or sport psychology counselor) conducting the interview understands the nature of the injury. This includes a working knowledge of the associated physical restrictions, the goals of treatment and rehabilitation, and the probable prognosis for return to sport. A comprehensive understanding of athletic injury is helpful because the psychosocial and physical repercussions of injury are closely intertwined. Emphasizing that the physical aspects of injury must be understood by the interviewer does not mean that the interviewer needs to personally conduct the physical assessment. However, to fully comprehend the injured athlete's experience, there must be communication between all members of the athlete's sports medicine team.

This chapter provides a guide for sports medicine practitioners (SMP) who wish to conduct a psychosocial assessment of the injured athlete. Several psychosocial assessment tools are discussed in detail and some are included for the reader's convenience.

In the past decade, partly due to the universal rise in healthcare costs, there has been increased pressure on medical practitioners to justify the effectiveness or outcome of the interventions provided to injured athletes. To facilitate the process (for medical practitioners' caring for injured athletes), physical (objective) and performance (functional) measures of injury outcome are listed and can be integrated into the psychosocial (subjective) assessment process. Finally, a case study will demonstrate the assessment procedure used in several sports medicine centers.

Assessment of the injured athlete

The interview setting

Whether one assesses injured athletes in a sports medicine center or in a training room, it is important to conduct the interview in an environment conducive to decreasing the athlete's discomfort and establishing a positive athlete–medical practitioner relationship. To help build trust, it is ideal if the athlete and medical practitioner share the same workspace at a table, which will help avoid the 'power seat'. This can be achieved by using a round table with two chairs of equal size. Additionally, the office décor should be pleasant and relaxing.[15,16] A clock should be positioned so that both the medical practitioner and the athlete can easily view the time. Lastly, displayed sport pictures and books help to convey an 'athletic' atmosphere, making the athlete feel more at ease.

To help build the athlete–medical practitioner relationship and show respect to the injured athlete, the environment should be free from distractions. Privacy is essential as athletes must feel free to express their true feelings without fear of being embarrassed or ridiculed. Because private office space is often at a premium, a quiet corner of a cafeteria, lounge, or a corner of the gym can be utilized. Ideally, the medical practitioner interviewer should 'hold' phone calls, turn his or her pager off, and have a sign outside the office door indicating that an interview is in session.

The assessment interview should be conducted with only the injured athlete in attendance. When parents, coaches, or significant others are present, no matter how well intentioned they are, too often the medical practitioner hears from everyone except the injured athlete. Furthermore, the assessment interview is one of the few opportunities the injured athlete has to be alone with a healthcare provider, and a very different response is frequently obtained than what might have been said in the presence of others. Injured athletes are typically more comfortable discussing feelings openly when there is no audience, and thus they have no need to conceal their emotions.

Timing of the assessment

Because the emotional response is so closely related to the physical diagnosis or the patient's perception of the injury, the assessment is more meaningful if it is conducted after the injury has been diagnosed. Therefore, in a sports medicine center, the psychosocial assessment of the injured athlete should take place after the injury has been diagnosed and the initial rehabilitation regimen has been discussed. The emotional response to injury parallels the athlete's rating of perceived recovery[4,12] and varies according to the injury diagnosis.[30] For example, a freshman softball player was injured during the first quarter of her softball season. When initially examined, the preliminary diagnosis was of a labial tear to her right shoulder, which would likely require surgery to correct. She learned, 3 weeks later, that she would not require surgery as she had only mild shoulder instability.[30] Because, in this case, the psychosocial assessment was conducted before the final diagnosis had been made, the initial interventions introduced were inappropriate. The emphasis at this time was spent on alleviating her surgical anxiety. The final diagnosis, however, confirmed that surgery was unnecessary. Thus, the interventions needed were related to her progressive strengthening program, which included goal-setting and guided mental imagery to help her focus on the specific shoulder muscles targeted for rehabilitation.

In the event that an athlete experiences a devastating injury (defined by the severity of the injury, timing of the injury relative to the sport season, other major life stress,[19,20,33] and an inadequate social support system),[18,20,21] it may be appropriate to see the athlete before the physical diagnosis has been made (i.e. MRI, bone scan, etc. may still be pending). The purpose of this preliminary session is to allow the athlete to make a connection and feel he or she is understood and supported. Such a session is not usually effective as an assessment interview because it is based on conjecture as opposed to facts. For example, if the injured skier introduced at the beginning of this chapter had been interviewed within 24 hours of the injury, it would not have been decided whether the injury was a transitory cord shock or a permanent spinal cord injury. This important distinction determines whether the skier returns to life's activities as an able-bodied participant or as a physically challenged athlete.

In a busy sports medicine practice, the interview process comprising the assessment, forming an impression, making a care plan, providing initial interventions, and arranging for a subsequent evaluation or follow-up, must all take place in approximately 1 hour.

Assessment etiquette

When first meeting the injured athlete, the medical practitioner should make eye contact, shake hands, facilitate introductions, and describe the purpose or goals of the interview as well as his or her qualifications for conducting the interview. It is important to make the athlete feel as physically and psychologically comfortable as possible. For instance, it may be appropriate to ask the athlete if he or she would feel more comfortable with the injured limb elevated. Ideally, prior to the interview the medical practitioner will have reviewed the medical record and be knowledgeable about the details of the athlete's injury.

Primary assessment tool used to measure the impact of injury

Rationale for ERAIQ

The interview process can be facilitated by using a psychosocial assessment form to guide the medical practitioner and the injured athlete through the assessment process. The Emotional Response of Athletes to Injury Questionnaire or ERAIQ[34-36] (see Appendix A) is a blueprint for the comprehensive assessment of the injured athlete. Questions are open-ended and the medical practitioner interviewer can probe areas of concern in more depth. Although the ERAIQ does not have established psychometric properties, it was developed from scores of clinical interviews with injured athletes and is integrated with the Wiese-Bjornstal and Smith model[35] (see Chapter 1 for details about this model). The ERAIQ has been published in various formats and is used by these authors on a daily basis to conduct assessments of injured athletes.[16,36]

The ERAIQ permits the medical practitioner to ask general, safe, but important questions before focusing on the core of the measure, namely the athlete's emotional response to injury. Trust is established as the medical practitioner asks the injured athlete about his or her dreams, preferred activities, reasons for participation in sport, perception of the injury, athletic identity, timing, characteristics of injury, impact of the injury on goals and sources of pressure, life stress, and social support prior to questions regarding the athlete's emotional response to injury. Coping strategies and abilities are assessed via questions about preferred activities, reasons for participating in sport and exercise, accepting responsibility for their injury and rehabilitation, and tolerating pain. The ERAIQ interview progresses through the athlete's perceived percentage of recovery, fear of re-injury, optimism, and knowledge of the prescribed rehabilitation exercises. See ref. 37 for an account of the development of the ERAIQ, or refs 5, 10, and 13 for a description of its use in other sports medicine settings.

Impression of the injured athlete

After reviewing the information obtained using the ERAIQ, an impression can be formed of the injured athlete's emotional status. To form the impression, the medical practitioner must decide, based on the injured athlete's affect (i.e. facial expression, tone of voice, energy level, posture, and eye contact), emotional response, and scores assigned to depression, tension, and anger, whether to quantify the athlete's depression or mood disturbance or to learn more about the nature and severity of other problems that have been detected. Figure 2.1 shows a flow chart of the assessment process. The impression categories depicted are simply a taxonomy used in our sports medicine center to guide the medical practitioner to appropriate interventions.

Because the Profile of Mood States (POMS)[38] (referred to in Fig. 2.1) has subscales for depression, tension, and anger (the three emotions identified most often on the ERAIQ) it is the psychological instrument often selected to quantify the injured athlete's total mood disturbance (TMD).

Before discussing the POMS and other complementary assessment tools in-depth, the process of referral, suggested in Fig. 2.1, for impression categories 3 and 4 is discussed.

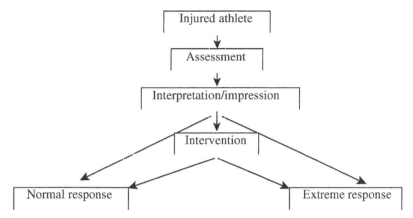

Fig. 2.1 This flow chart depicts the process of assessing the athlete, forming an impression, and planning interventions, which may also include referral of the athlete. (Reprinted with permission from Ray, R. (1999). *Counseling in sports medicine*, p. 89. Human Kinetics, Champaign, IL.)

Referral of the injured athlete

The need to refer an injured athlete for more in-depth psychological or psychiatric assessment will vary depending on the education, qualifications, and expertise of the medical practitioner who conducts the assessment interview. In some sports medicine centers, mental health professionals (e.g. sport psychologists, clinical psychologists, or psychiatrists) who have a special interest in athletes are available for consultation.[15]

In the impression depicted in Fig. 2.1 category 3 (minor injury, exaggerated consequences, little social support, poor coping skills), an in-depth clinical assessment may be required to identify psychosocial features exacerbating the response to injury. Athletes may fear sport participation and may experience pressure from others to participate. Although many athletes in this category can often be assisted by the sport psychologist, others may require a prompt clinical assessment to ensure they do not develop problems such as dysfunctional gaits, malingering, or chronic pain syndrome.

In the Impression 4 situation (injury is severe; consequences are grave; despite strong social support and good coping skills, the athlete is still depressed) the injured athlete is appropriately depressed, as the injury is severe and the consequences are grim. Occasionally, despite the psychological skills training strategies introduced and the athlete's own social support system and coping skills, a referral is necessary for assessment and treatment of clinical depression.

Medical practitioners should identify mental health professionals who are helpful, interested, and willing to see injured athletes in the event that a referral is needed.

Rationale for the POMS

The POMS[38] quantifies mood-state scores for each of the six subscales measuring tension, depression, anger, vigor, fatigue, and confusion. A total mood disturbance score (TMD) is calculated by adding the negative mood scales (i.e., depression, anger, fatigue, and confusion) and subtracting the positive mood scale (vigor). It is a 65-item, 5-point Likert scale requiring the subject to rate adjectives. It is suitable for persons with at least a 7th grade education (usually 12 or 13 years of age) and takes 3–5 minutes to complete. A sample of questions asked on the POMS is provided in Appendix B.

Weinberg and Gould[39] (p. 40 therein) recommended that the POMS be used to monitor the emotional response of athletes to injury.[4,9,12,13,23,40] Although the POMS was not specifically developed for athletes, there are normative data for college-aged students. Injured athletes in our practice range from approximately 16 to 25 years of age. Therefore, college normative data (see ref. 38, p. 28 therein) are comparable to the ages of most injured athletes. The POMS has been used extensively with athletes, resulting in a mental health model used to predict athletic success.[41–44] It is recommended that the POMS be used in situations where each athlete serves as his/her own point of reference rather than being compared to norms.[40] Most athletes with minor injuries have less TMD than college norms, whereas seriously injured athletes often have higher scores on depression, tension, anger, fatigue, and confusion, and lower vigor than college norms.[4,9,13,40] Recently, normative scores[45] have been determined based on international ($n = 622$), club ($n = 638$), and recreational ($n = 836$) athletic samples. These athletes reported a more positive mood state than college norms, who were used as a basis for comparison in earlier studies on injured athletes.

The 'iceberg profile' in sport[42] depicts the normative graph, or positive mood state of non-injured athletes. During the assessment interview, the injured athlete is often shown the positive mood state graph (represented by low tension, depression, anger, fatigue, and confusion, and high vigor) that he or she might have enjoyed prior to injury as an exercising and competitive athlete. The athlete's current, postinjury POMS profile is then graphed alongside the normative, positive mood state. The seriously injured athlete's postinjury scores usually reflect marked TMD. Depression most often occurs in a reciprocal relationship with vigor. For example, when depression is high, vigor is usually low, which may negatively impact on rehabilitation behavior.

Measures of internal consistency (validity), which detect how effectively the individual items within the six mood scales predict the factor they are designed to predict, are near 0.90 or above. The POMS tests, manual, and scoring key can be ordered from EDITS in San Diego, California by writing or calling Educational and Industrial Testing Services.

Frequently, depression, self-esteem, pain, and overly invested athletic identity[8] have an impact on rehabilitation behaviors[23]and thus need to be assessed. Some of the complementary assessment tools used to address these problems are discussed below.

Complementary assessment tools

The Sports Medicine Observation Code (SMOC)

This code can be used in situations where the medical practitioner questions whether a lack of physical progress is related to the injured athlete's adherence to rehabilitation.[46] The SMOC allows the medical practitioner to objectively quantify the frequency and the time that injured athletes spend doing rehabilitation exercises.

There are 11 rehabilitation behavior categories defined in the SMOC,[46] which include active rehabilitation, initial treatment, attending-related, attending-unrelated, interaction-related, interaction-unrelated, waiting, initial diagnosis, preventive treatment, maintenance, non-activity, unrelated activity, and exclusion (see Appendix C for definitions). The observer can either record a behavior at the end of a given time-frame (time-sampling) or the primary behavior (interval recording) occurring within a given time interval (i.e., 10 seconds). Such observations may be helpful when the medical practitioner has prescribed the therapy or is busy with other injured athletes. Sometimes a lack of rehabilitation progress is not related to the time or effort spent on rehabilitation exercises (as measured on the SMOC), but is impeded by the physical pain experienced, which may need to be assessed.

The Sport Inventory for Pain (SIP)

The Sport Inventory for Pain (SIP)[47] was developed to predict pain-coping responses in injured athletes. The SIP uses a 5-point Likert scale to assess five pain subscales: coping (eight items), cognitive (five items), avoidance (four items), catastrophizing (four items), and body awareness (four items) (see Appendix D). Collectively these subscales yield a composite score, indicative of the injured athlete's ability to cope with pain. Reliability measures range from 0.61 to 0.88. Similarly, test–retest correlations range from 0.69 to 0.88.

The SIP did not change significantly when administered at four data-collection periods to patients having anterior cruciate-ligament reconstruction.[5,48] Recall that the SIP does not measure changes in the amount of pain experienced, but instead measures the athlete's ability to cope with pain. Occasionally, the athlete is not experiencing significant pain, but may fail to progress well in rehabilitation because of skepticism about the value of rehabilitation exercises.

The Sports Injury Rehabilitation Beliefs Survey (SIRBS)

The SIRBS is a helpful inventory for detecting the degree to which the injured athlete believes in or values the prescribed rehabilitation program.[49] Because beliefs or values are the foundation of our thoughts (cognitions) and so direct our emotional responses and rehabilitation behaviors,[23,35] an assessment of beliefs about the value of rehabilitation therapy and exercising is appropriate.

The SIRBS contains 19 questions on a Likert scale, ranging from 1 (very strongly disagree) to 7 (very strongly agree)[49]. Questions pertain to injury recovery, recurrence, perceived recovery, potential for reinjury, perceived efficacy, competency, and the perceived severity of the injury (see Appendix E). The inventory has five subscales that relate to: susceptibility, treatment efficacy, self-efficacy, value of rehabilitation, and perceived severity.[49] In the event that subscale scores are lower than optimal, the medical practitioner will know which beliefs or values must be targeted to provide additional education for the injured athlete. Athletes may progress poorly in rehabilitation because they are either not sufficiently identified with sport (i.e. apathetic) or, conversely, they may be devastated because of a strong athletic identity.

Athletic Identity Measurement Scale (AIMS)

The purpose of the AIMS is to identify athletes who may be overly invested in sport as a result of a strong athletic identity. Athletic identity consists of thoughts, feelings, behaviors, and social effects unique to individuals who identify with the athlete role.[8] When an athlete's focus is solely on sport, athletic identity may be too strong. Those athletes who overly identify with sport are more vulnerable to emotional and social difficulties in the event of an injury.[8] The AIMS has 10 questions answered on a Likert scale of 1 (strongly agree) to 7 (strongly disagree) and the highest score possible is 70 (see Appendix F). Scoring is such that 50–70 indicates the athlete is highly or exclusively identified with sport; 31–49 reflects moderate identity; 7–30 is indicative of a very low athletic identity. This measure can be administered if the injured athlete is markedly depressed and it is suspected that he or she is overly identified with sport. Depending on the athlete's goals, dreams, and level of participation, the AIMS helps to identify athletes who overidentify with sport so that strategies can be put in place to help them gain a broader perspective on life. The results of the AIMS are interpreted in context with the impact and the consequences of the athlete's injury. It may be necessary to counsel the athlete on career-development, advanced education, financial planning, and social identity issues to help facilitate their adjustment to injury.[50]

Other complementary assessments

The additional complementary assessment measures listed in Table 2.1 can be selected for use based on identification of a problem from the assessment interview or on a lack of progress in rehabilitation, which may be detected later. For example, although a decrease between pre- and postinjury self-esteem was not significant in a 13 team study,[40] lowered self-esteem was reported in injured runners compared to their non-injured counterparts.[9] The Rosenberg Self-esteem Inventory[51] or the Tennessee Self-concept Scale[52] can be administered (see Table 2.1) if low self-esteem is suspected.

All the complementary measures listed in Table 2.1 have established validity and reliability with the exception of the ERAIQ. Also, the Rehabilitation Adherence Questionnaire (RAQ)[27] and the Sport Injury Survey (SIS)[31] lack reliability.

The primary and complementary assessment measures, while helpful in quantifying the areas of concern to the injured athlete and the medical practitioner, are only helpful when they are integrated with information regarding other obstacles or barriers likely to impede optimal rehabilitation.

Identification of barriers

It is believed that exercise compliance or adherence to rehabilitation is necessary to achieve the desired outcome (full return to sport). Although measuring adherence is fraught with difficulty, adherence to rehabilitation exercises (e.g. because of a reconstructed knee or shoulder) is clearly extremely important. For example, joint pain is more pronounced when muscles have not been strengthened properly postinjury. Athletes who have had their anterior cruciate ligament (ACL) reconstructed may lose up to 1.5 inches of girth size in the quadricep muscle. Muscles will not return to their preinjury status without physical work and compliance to the rehabilitation exercises prescribed.

The best measure of adherence is simply whether or not the fundamental and objective goals of rehabilitation are being achieved. Although this may be unfair since rehabilitation goals may be met more easily by some than

Table 1 Complementary psychological assessments

Instrument	Author/year (ref. no.)	Purpose	Length of questionnaire
Athletic Identity Measurement Scale (AIMS)	Brewer, Van Raalte, and Linder 1993 (8)	Examines athlete's role identification	10 items
Beck Depression Inventory (BDI)	Beck, Ward, Mendelson, Mock, and Erbaugh 1961 (53)	Assesses depression symptom severity	21 items
Coping with Health Injuries and Problems Scale (CHIP)	Endler, Parker, and Summerfeldt 1993 (54)	Identifies perceived coping for a variety of health problems	34 items
Emotional Responses of Athletes to Injury Questionnaire (ERAIQ)	Smith, Scott, O'Fallon, and Young 1990 (4)	Identifies emotional response to injury	25 items
Locus of Control in Rehabilitation Scale (LCRS)	Duda, Smart, and Tappe 1989 (24)	Assesses athlete's perceived control over rehabilitation	9 items
Minnesota Multiphasic Personality Inventory (MMPI)	Butcher, Dahlstrom, Graham, Tellegen, and Kaemmer 1987 (55)	Measures and detects major psychological and psychiatric illnesses	Approximately 650 questions
Physical Self-profile (PSP)	Fox and Corbin 1989 (56)	Examines physical self-perceptions	Five, 6-item perception subscales
Profile of Mood States (POMS)	McNair, Lorr, and Droppleman 1992 (38)	Identifies feelings and mood states	65 adjectives
Rehabilitation Adherence Questionnaire (RAQ)	Fischer, Domm, and Wuest 1988 (27)	Examines factors that relate to rehabilitation adherence	40 items
Sports Attitude Inventory (SAI)	Willis 1982 (57)	Assesses competitive motives in sport	40 items
Sports Injury Clinic Athlete Satisfaction Scale (SICASS)	Taylor and May 1995 (32)	Examines perceived satisfaction with sports medicine care	13 items
Sport Injury Rehabilitation Adherence Scale (SIRAS)	Brewer, Van Raalte, Petitpas, Sklar, and Ditmar 1995 (22)	Measures adherence during sport injury rehabilitation	3 items
Sports Injury Rehabilitation Beliefs Survey (SIRBS)	Taylor and May 1996 (49)	Assesses athletes' rehabilitation beliefs	18 items
Sports Injury Survey (SIS)	Ievleva and Orlick 1991 (31)	Identifies characteristics of the healing process	25 questions
Sports Inventory for Pain (SIP)	Meyers, Bourgeois, Stewart, and LeUnes 1992 (47)	Examines strategies used to cope with pain	25 items
Rosenberg Self-esteem Inventory (RSEI)	Rosenberg 1968 (51)	Assesses global self-esteem	10 items
Tennessee Self-concept Scale (TSCS)	Roid and Fitts 1988 (52)	Measures self-perceptions	100 items

others, the clinically relevant question relates to the progress being made. Progress made at specific 'milestones' during rehabilitation assures the sports medicine team that the desired recovery outcome will be achieved.[58] Because 'progress milestones' are emphasized during rehabilitation, assessment of psychosocial and physical outcomes at specific times is important. Although various measures of adherence (e.g. perceived effort, appropriate attitude toward rehabilitation) are of interest, the emphasis of rehabilitation is becoming increasingly 'functional by orientation'[58] with fewer sessions supervised and more rehabilitation being the athlete's responsibility to complete at home.[59] Athletes are now being cleared for return to sport much earlier than in the past. As such, the comprehensive assessment process must evolve and keep pace with the dynamic nature of the clinical practice.

Trend toward integrated assessment (quality of life)

Barriers to rehabilitation may relate to psychosocial influences such as lack of motivation, lack of perceived value or belief in the rehabilitation exercises, and fear of reinjury. Barriers to rehabilitation also include physical factors such as excessive swelling, muscle inhibition, reflex sympathetic dystrophy, or infection, which may occur despite compliance to rehabilitation. Although these complications rarely occur, physical barriers may require that the injured athlete plateaus until these problems are medically controlled. Such barriers are frustrating to both the injured athlete and the medical practitioner, and so may require additional psychosocial assessment and intervention[25] until resolved.

Medical practitioner professionals are interested in subjective (psychosocial), objective, and functional outcomes. These three dimensions of outcome are closely related. For example, an excellent objective outcome measure, such as full range of motion, is of no value if the patient cannot later use the limb or joint without pain or functional limitations. Clearly, an ideal surgical or non-surgical intervention with appropriate rehabilitation will demonstrate improvement in all three spheres.

Psychosocial and physical outcomes are depicted in the center of the Wiese-Bjornstal–Smith Model (1993) (see Chapter 1) because they are the target of all rehabilitation interventions. Few studies have reported on the injured athlete's objective,[10,29,48] subjective,[60] and functional outcomes.

Quality of Life (QOL) is a state of physical, mental, and social well-being. A comprehensive assessment, appropriate to the injured athlete, contains measures of these three spheres. In addition to the ERAIQ and POMS (which are most often used in the first week or two following injury), other subjective measures of QOL can be included in the assessment interview with the injured athlete, or administered prior to the athlete's return to sport.

Table 2.2   Subjective measures

Instrument	Author/year (ref. no.)	Purpose	Length of questionnaire
MOS 36-Item Short-Form Health Survey (SF-36)	Ware and Sherbourne 1992 (61)	General health status	36 items
Oswestry Disability Index (ODI)	Fairbank, Davies, Couper, and O'Brien 1980 (62)	Patient's self-assessment of back pain	10 items
Quality of Life for Chronic Anterior Cruciate Ligament (ACL-QOL)	Mohtadi 1998 (63)	Quality of life of patients with chronic ACL deficiencies	32 items
Subjective Knee Score Questionnaire	Wilk, Romaniello, Soscia, Arrigo, and Andrews 1994 (64)	Symptoms and sport activities related to ACL reconstruction	8 categories

Although not all are specific to the injured athlete, they can provide information about the athlete's perception of 'wellness'.

Subjective measures

Subjective measures are particularly helpful as assessment tools if administered prior to surgery or prior to a non-surgical rehabilitation program and again before return to sport. Ideally, changes in the subscales, particularly for activity, will reflect improved status and the injured athletes' psychosocial readiness to return to sport or exercise.

Even though a generic, subjective quality-of-life assessment indicates life satisfaction, medical practitioners cannot assume that improved QOL is attributable to a specific surgical or non-surgical intervention. For example, an individual's QOL might improve 60% because of a romantic involvement thereby obscuring the fact that shoulder function and pain may not have improved following the recent surgery.

Of interest to medical practitioners (because of the number of anterior cruciate ligament (ACL)-deficient patients seen in sports medicine centers), is the ACL-QOL (see Table 2.2).[63] The ACL-QOL is a psychosocial (subjective), objective, and functional outcome measure specific to anterior cruciate ligament-deficient patients, which enables investigators to attribute improvement to ACL-specific surgical or non-surgical interventions. The ACL-QOL[63] has five subscales relating to physical knee symptoms, work issues, recreation and sport activity, social/emotional factors, and lifestyle issues. The ACL-QOL can measure the perceived benefits of a surgical ACL reconstruction, appropriate in the treatment of ACL deficiency in high-demand sport athletes, or the benefit of non-surgical rehabilitation, which is appropriate to athletes involved in less physically demanding sports.

Objective measures

Decisions on whether to proceed with a surgical or a non-surgical intervention are based on subjective and objective measures. The degree of ligamentous laxity and effusion in a joint, or the lack of flexion or extension are examples of objective measures. Furthermore, progress is initially determined based on achievement of objective measures.

Successful objective outcomes in strength, stability, and mobility (to reduce the risk of subsequent injury) are essential if the athlete seeks to return to preinjury status. It is also pertinent to ensure that the joint has the desired functional outcome that convinces athletes that rehabilitation is complete and they are physically and psychologically ready to return to sport.

Functional outcomes

A golf swing, a pitch thrown at a specific velocity, and a biomechanically correct tennis serve are examples of upper-body, functional outcome measures.

The vertical leap, agility drills, hops, skips, lunges, and sprints are lower-body, functional outcome measures that assure the injured athlete that the surgical procedure, rehabilitation exercises, and treatment modalities were worthwhile. The following case study shows the integration of various assessment measures appropriate to the psychosocial evaluation of a 17-year-old injured athlete.

Case study

James is a 17-year-old baseball, basketball, and track and field high-school athlete who tore his anterior cruciate ligament, medial meniscus, and the medial collateral ligament while playing in the state high-school basketball championships during his Junior year. A few major giving-way (buckling) episodes convinced James and his athletic trainer to seek a referral to a sports medicine center. After an evaluation with an orthopedic surgeon, James was referred to a sport psychologist for a psychosocial assessment and the appropriate preoperative (ACL reconstruction) patient education.

James and his sport psychologist used the ERAIQ to assess his psychosocial response to injury. During the interview, it was discovered that his dream goal in life was to play professional baseball and that he participated in sports primarily for competition, fun, and self-discipline. After the injury, he felt pressure from his coaches, peers, team-mates, and the citizens in his small town. He felt he had 'let the team down'.[65] Even though James had a strong social support network, he felt depressed and sad. On the ERAIQ, James ranked depression 12, frustration 11, anger 10, frightened 9, and helpless 8, where the highest possible ranking score is 12.

After assessing the emotional response to injury, the sport psychologist formed an impression. James fitted the criteria for category 2 (see Fig. 2.1). However, his usual sources of social support unintentionally made him feel badly, hinting that the team would not be successful without him. Because of high depression on the ERAIQ, the POMS was administered. James's tension score was 12, depression 33, anger 27, vigor 3, fatigue 25, and confusion 22 (Fig. 2.2). This result on the POMS (marked as preoperatively on Fig. 2.2) reflects marked TMD and depleted energy resources (low vigor)—a worrisome situation.

Although the preoperative depression score was not as high as that experienced by injured athletes who have attempted suicide,[6] because of his investment in sport,[8] his flat affect, and his worry about letting the team down,[21] the questions used to assess suicidal ideation were asked. James and his parents were asked to call the counselor in the event that depression increased prior to his surgical ACL reconstruction scheduled for 2 weeks later. Fortunately, James focused on factors under his control, such as preparing for his surgery. As a result, his depression did not increase.

After his ACL reconstruction, James and his counselor charted his progress and noted the decrease in TMD (marked as 2 days' postoperatively in Fig. 2.2), which, as discussed, usually parallels the athlete's perception that recovery or progress in rehabilitation is occurring.[4,12,28,29] Subjective improvement was noted on James' ACL-QOL scores between pre- and postoperative evaluations.[60,63] The ACL-QOL was administered to James preoperatively, then postoperatively at 6 months, 1 year, and 2 years. The results for the four sequential measurements for the total ACL-QOL score and the scores for the individual subscales are provided in Table 2.3.

This case study was used to illustrate the psychosocial assessment of James, integrating the ERAIQ, POMS, and, because of the nature of the injury, the ACL-QOL. The greatly improved mood state profile 6 months' postoperatively was supported by the improved ACL-QOL scores in all subscales. Notable, however, is the improved activity subscale noted in sport activity between 6 months and 2 years. Two years after surgery, James had regained the confidence necessary to be a highly functioning, competitive athlete.

Table 3   Quality of Life (ACL-QOL)

Time of evaluation	Total score	Symptoms and physical complaints (*n* = 5)	Work-related concerns (*n* = 4)	Sport activity (*n* = 12)	Lifestyle (*n* = 6)	Emotional/ social concerns (*n* = 5)
Preop.	38.3	53.6	40.8	21.6	51.7	45
6 months postop.	58.8	65.6	70.8	45	76.3	54.8
1 year postop.	79.3	67.6	78.5	60.8	78	73.2
2 years postop.	92.8	86.6	97.8	92.5	95.3	92.6

n, Number of items on each subscale.
Scores are out of a possible 100 points (high scores are desirable).
ACL, anterior cruciate ligament.

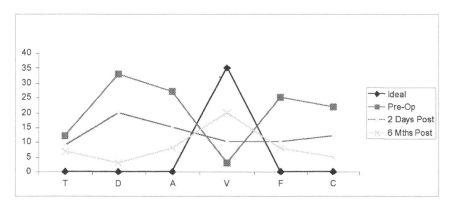

Fig. 2.2   Graph of the Profile of Mood States subscale scores following anterior cruciate ligament injury (pre- and postoperatively) contrasted with the 'iceberg' profile (a mood state described for non-injured athletes.[42]

Conclusions

In this chapter, the authors have provided the rationale and suggested a procedure for conducting a psychosocial assessment of an injured athlete. Modifications in the interview process described can be made to accommodate individual differences based on the injured athlete's situation and the medical practitioner's needs, experience, education, and preferences. Furthermore, in addition to conducting an assessment of the injured athlete, this chapter also emphasized the importance of assessing the effectiveness of all interventions provided by the medical practitioner team. Interventions must be evaluated comprehensively so their effect on the athlete's psychosocial and physical outcome can be determined. Only when injured athletes are fully rehabilitated, have returned functionally to their desired level of activity, and have demonstrated satisfaction can it be said that a successful outcome of either surgical or non-surgical interventions has been achieved.[63]

Although the psychosocial impact of injury is not usually serious for the majority of injured athletes, the magnitude of the response experienced by some of the more seriously injured athletes justifies the assessment process. Meeting the injured athlete, expressing interest and concern, and learning about the correlates of injury help to foster a therapeutic relationship between the medical practitioner and the injured athlete. This relationship provides an excellent point of departure for the introduction of appropriate interventions[15,21,25,30,31,34,65] that enhance the rehabilitation process.

Acknowledgments

The authors would like to express their appreciation for the Johannson-Gund endowment, to Ms Heather Peters, Mr Scott Kronebusch, Mr Joshua Holmes, Mr Tim McLean (P.T., MS), Mr Phil Orte (P.T.), Mr Dave Schroeder (P.T.), Mr Lynn Duncan (P.T., MS, ATC), Mr Dave Krause (P.T.), Ms Connie Bruce, Ms Patricia Erwin (Reference Librarian at the Mayo Clinic), Ms Pam Darcy, and Mr Chad Rypstra for their assistance with this chapter.

References

1. Meeuwisse, W. H. and Fowler, P. J. (1988). Frequency and predictability of sports injuries in intercollegiate athletics. *Canadian Journal of Sport Sciences*, **13**, 35–42.
2. Kraus, J. F. and Conroy, C. (1984). Mortality and morbidity from injuries in sports and recreation. *Annual Review of Public Health*, **5**, 163–92.
3. Crossman, J., Gluck, L., and Jamieson, J. (1995). The emotional response of injured athletes. *New Zealand Journal of Sports Medicine*, **23**, 1–2.

4. Smith, A. M., Scott, S. G., O'Fallon, W., and Young, M. L. (1990). The emotional responses of athletes to injury. *Mayo Clinic Proceedings*, **65**, 38–50.
5. Morrey, M. A., Stuart, M. J., Smith, A. M. and Wiese-Bjornstal, D. M. (1999). A longitudinal examination of an athlete's emotional and cognitive responses to anterior cruciate ligament injury. *Clinical Journal of Sports Medicine*, 9, 63–9.
6. Smith, A. M. and Milliner, E. K. (1994). Injured athletes and the risk of suicide. *Journal of Athletic Training*, **29**, 337–41.
7. Asken, M. J. (1999). Counseling athletes with catastrophic injury and illness. In *Counseling in Sports Medicine* (ed. R. Ray, and D. M. Wiese-Bjornstal), pp. 293–309. Human Kinetics, Champaign, IL.
8. Brewer, B. W., Van Raalte, J. L., and Linder, D. E. (1993). Athletic identity: Hercules muscles or Achilles heel? *International of Sport Psychology*, **24**, 237–54.
9. Chan, C. S. and Grossman, H. Y. (1988). Psychological effects of running loss on consistent runners. *Perceptual and Motor Skills*, **66**, 875–83.
10. LaMott, E. E. (1994). The anterior cruciate ligament injured athlete: The psychological process. Unpublished PhD dissertation. University of Minnesota, Minneapolis, MN.
11. Leddy, M. H., Lambert, M. J., and Ogles, B. M. (1994). Psychological consequences of athletic injury among high level competition. *Research Quarterly for Exercise and Sport*, **65**, 349–54.
12. McDonald, S. A. and Hardy, C. J. (1990). Affective response patterns of the injured athlete: An exploratory analysis. *The Sports Psychologist*, 4, 261–74.
13. Pearson, L. and Jones, G. (1992). Emotional effects of sports injuries: Implications for physiotherapists. *Physiotherapy*, **78**, 762–70.
14. Quackenbush, N. and Crossman, J. (1994). Injured athletes: A study of emotional responses. *Journal of Sport Behavior*, **17**, 178–87.
15. Wiese-Bjornstal, D. M. and Smith, A. M. (1993). Counseling strategies for enhanced recovery of injured athletes within a team approach. In *Psychological bases of sports injuries* (ed. D. Pargman), pp. 149–182. Fitness Information Technology, Morgantown, WV.
16. Smith, A. M. (1999). Assessing athletes through individual interview. In *Counseling in sports medicine* (ed. R. Ray, and D. M. Wiese-Bjornstal), pp. 00–00. Human Kinetics, Champaign, IL.
17. Brewer, B. W., Linder, D. E., and Phelps, C. M. (1995). Situational correlates of emotional adjustment to athletic injury. *Clinical Journal of Sport Medicine*, **5**, 241–5.
18. Hardy, C. J., Burke, K. L., and Crace, R. K. (1999). Social support and injury: A framework for social support-based interventions with injured athletes. In *Psychological bases of sport injury* (2nd edn) (ed. D. Pargman), pp. 121–144. Fitness Information Technology, Morgantown, WV.
19. Andersen, M. B. and Williams, J. M. (1988). A model of stress and athletic injury: Prediction and prevention. *Journal of Sport and Exercise Psychology*, **10**, 294–306.

20. Smith, R. E., Smoll, F. L., and Ptacek, J. T. (1990). Conjunctive moderator variables in vulnerability and resiliency research: Life stress, social support, and coping skills and adolescent sport injuries. *Journal of Personality and Social Psychology*, **58**, 360–70.

21. Udry, E. M. (1997). Coping and social support among injured athletes following surgery. *Journal of Sport and Exercise Psychology*, **19**, 71–90.

22. Brewer, B. W., Van Raalte, J. L., Petitpas, A. J., Sklar, J. H., and Ditmar, T. D. (1995). A brief measure of adherence during sport injury rehabilitation sessions. *Journal of Applied Sport Psychology*, **7**, S44. [Abstract]

23. Daly, J. M., Brewer, B. W., VanRaalte, J. L., Petipas, A. J., and Sklar, J. H. (1995). Cognitive appraisal, emotional adjustment, and adherence to rehabilitation following knee surgery. *Journal of Sport Rehabilitation*, **4**, 22–30.

24. Duda, J. L., Smart, A. E., and Tappe, M. K. (1989). Predictors of adherence in rehabilitation of athletic injuries: An application of personal investment theory. *Journal of Sport and Exercise Psychology*, **11**, 367–81.

25. Durso Cupal, D. (1998). Psychological interventions in sport injury. Prevention and rehabilitation. *Journal of Applied Sport Psychology*, **10**, 103–23.

26. Evans, L. and Hardy, L. (1995). Sport injury and grief responses. A review. *Journal of Sport and Exercise Psychology*, **17**, 227–45.

27. Fischer, C. A., Domm, M. A., and Wuest, D. A. (1988). Adherence to sports-injury rehabilitation programs. *The Physician and Sportsmedicine*, **16**, 47–51.

28. Grove, J. R. and Bianco, T. (1999). Personality correlates of psychological processes during injury rehabilitation. In *Psychological bases of sports injuries* (2nd edn) (ed. D. Pargman), pp. 89–110. Fitness Information Technology, Morgantown, WV.

29. Grove, J. R. (1993). Personality and injury rehabilitation among sport performers. In *Psychological bases of sports injuries* (ed. D. Pargman), pp. 99–120. Fitness Information Technology, Morgantown, WV.

30. Hartman, A. D. and Finch, L. M. (1999). The use of goal setting to facilitate social support for injured athletes. Unpublished Master's thesis. Western Illinois University, IL.

31. Ievleva, L. and Orlick, T. (1991). Mental links to enhanced healing: An exploratory study. *The Sport Psychologist*, **5**, 25–40.

32. Taylor, A. H. and May, S. (1995). Development of a sports injury clinic athlete satisfaction scale for auditing patient perceptions. *Physiotherapy Theory and Practice*, **11**, 231–8.

33. Smith, A. M., Stuart, M. J., Wiese-Bjornstal, D. M., and Gunnon, C. (1997). Predictors of injury in ice hockey players: A multivariate, multidisciplinary approach. *The American Journal of Sportsmedicine*, **25**, 500–7.

34. Smith, A. M., Scott, S. G., and Wiese, D. M. (1990). The psychological effects of sports injuries: coping. *Sports Medicine*, **9**, 352–69.

35. Wiese-Bjornstal, D. M., Smith, A. M., Shaffer, S. M., and Morrey, M. A.

(1998). An integrated model of response to sport injury: Psychological and sociological dynamics. *Journal of Applied Sports Psychology*, **10**, 46–69.

36. Smith, A. M. (1996). Psychological impact of injuries in athletes. *Sports Medicine*, **22**, 391–405.

37. Smith, A. M. (1988). The emotional responses of athletes to injury. Unpublished Master's thesis. University of Minnesota, Minneapolis, MN.

38. McNair, D. M., Lorr, M., and Droppleman, L. F. (1992). *EDITS manual for the Profile of Mood States*. Educational and Industrial Testing Service, San Diego, CA.

39. Weinberg, R. S. and Gould, D. (1999). Personality and sport. In *Foundations of sport and exercise psychology* (2nd edn) (ed. R. S. Weinberg and D. Gould), pp. 40. Human Kinetics, Champaign, IL.

40. Smith, A. M., Stuart, M. J., Wiese-Bjornstal, D. M., Milliner, E. K., O'Fallon, W. J., and Crowson, C. S. (1993). Competitive athletes: Pre and post injury mood state and self-esteem. *Mayo Clinic Proceedings*, **68**, 939–47.

41. Morgan, W. P. (1979). Prediction of performance in athletics. In *Coach, athlete, and the sport psychologist* (ed. P. Klavora and J. V. Daniel), pp. 173–86. Human Kinetics, Champaign, IL.

42. Morgan, W. P. (1980). A test of champions. *Psychology Today*, **14**, 92–108.

43. Morgan, W. P., Brown, D. R., Raglin, J. S., O'Connor, P. J., and Ellickson, K. A. (1987). Psychological monitoring of overtraining and staleness. *British Journal of Sport Medicine*, **21**, 107–14.

44. Terry, P. C. (1995). The efficacy of mood state profiling with elite performers: A review and synthesis. *The Sport Psychologist*, **9**, 309–24.

45. Terry, P. C. and Lane, A. M. (2000). Normative values for the profile of mood states for use with athletic samples. *The Journal of Applied Sport Psychology*, **12**, 93–109.

46. Crossman, J. and Roch, J. (1991). An observational instrument for use in sports medicine clinics. *Canadian Journal of Physical Therapy*, April, 10–13.

47. Meyers, C., Bourgeois, A. E., Stewart, S., and LeUnes, A. (1992). Predicting pain responses in athletes: Development and assessment of the Sports Inventory for Pain. *Journal of Sport and Exercise Psychology*, **14**, 249–61.

48. Morrey, M. A. (1997). A longitudinal examination of emotional response, cognitive coping, and physical recovery among athletes undergoing anterior cruciate ligament reconstructive surgery. Unpublished PhD dissertation. University of Minnesota, Minneapolis, MN.

49. Taylor, A. H. and May, S. (1996). Threat and coping appraisal as determinants of compliance with sports injury rehabilitation: An application of protection motivation theory. *Journal of Sport Sciences*, **14**, 471–82.

50. Finnie, S. B. and Fischer, T. L. (1999). Learning life skills through hockey. In *Power play* (3rd edn) (ed. A. Smith), pp. 161–170. Athletic Guide Publishing, Flagler Beach, FL.

51. Rosenberg, M. (1968). *Society and the adolescent self-image*. Princeton University Press, Princeton, NJ.

52. Roid, G. H. and Fitts, W. (1988). *Tennessee Self-Concept Scale (TSCS): revised manual.* Western Psychological Services, Los Angeles, CA.

53. Beck, A. T., Ward, C. H., Mendelson, M., Mock, J., and Erbaugh, J. (1961). An inventory for measuring depression. *Archives of General Psychiatry*, **4**, 561–71.

54. Endler, N. S., Parker, J. D. A., and Summerfeldt, L. J. (1998). Coping with health problems: Developing a reliable and valid multidimensional measure. *Psychological Assessment*, **10**, 195–205.

55. Butcher, J. N., Dahlstrom, W. G., Graham, J. R., Tellegen, A., and Kaemmer, B. (1987). MMPI-2. *Minnesota Multiphasic Personality Inventory—2. Manual for administration for scoring.* University of Minnesota Press, Minneapolis, MN.

56. Fox, K. R. and Corbin, C. B. (1989). The physical self-perception profile: Development and preliminary validation. *Journal of Sport and Exercise Psychology*, **11**, 408–30.

57. Willis, J. D. (1982). Three scales to measure competition-related motives in sport. *Journal of Sport Psychology*, **4**, 338–53.

58. McLean, T. (1999). Validation of the costs of physical therapy by outcome based utilization analysis in the sports medicine center of the Mayo foundation. Unpublished Master's thesis. Cardinal Stritch University, Rochester, MN.

59. Fischer, D. A., Tewes, D. P., Boyd, J. L., Smith, J. P., and Quick, D. C. (1998). Home based rehabilitation for anterior cruciate ligament reconstruction. *Clinical Orthopedics and Related Research*, **347**, 194–9.

60. Smith, A. M., Stuart, M. J., Laskowski, E. R., Morrey, M. A., Worm, S. C., and Malo, S. A. (1999). A quality of life comparison of pre and post surgery anterior cruciate ligament reconstruction patients. *Presented at the Association for the Advancement of Applied Sport Psychology*, pp. 44, Banff, Alberta, Canada. JASP Abstracts, **12**, Supplement.

61. Ware, J. E. and Sherbourne, C. D. (1992). The MOS 36-item Short-Form Health Survey (SF-36): 1. Conceptual framework and item selection. *Medical Care*, **30**, 473–81.

62. Fairbank, J. C. T., Davies, J., Couper, J., and O'Brien, J. P. (1980). Oswestry disability questionnaire. *Physiotherapy*, **66**, 271–3.

63. Mohtadi, N. (1998). Development and validation of the quality of life outcome measure (questionnaire) for chronic anterior cruciate ligament deficiency. *The American Journal of Sports Medicine*, **26**, 350–9.

64. Wilk, K. E., Romaniello, W. T., Soscia, S. M., Arrigo, C. A., and Andrews, J. R. (1994). The relationship between subjective knee scores, isokinetic testing, and functional testing in the ACL-reconstructed knee. *Journal of Orthopaedic and Sports Physical Therapy*, **20**, 60–73.

65. Heil, J. (1999). The injured athlete. In *Emotions in sport* (ed. Y. L. Hanins), pp. 264–5. Human Kinetics, Champaign, IL.

Appendices to chapter 2

Appendix A

A

The Emotional Responses of Athletes To Injury Questionnaire

Name	Date
Address	Age D.O.B
City State Zip	Clinic #
Phone (H) (W)	Ht Wt

If you could be anything you wanted to be in life, what would your dream be?

List in order of preference the sports and activities that you participate in.
1   2
3   4

Why do you participate in sports? (10 = high, 0 = low)
...... Self-discipline ...... Stress management
...... Competition ...... Personal improvement
...... Socialization ...... Outlet of aggression
...... Fitness   ...... Weight management
...... Fun   ...... Other, i.e. well being

Would you describe yourself as an athlete? (circle)
     1   2   3   4   5
(absolutely not)   (absolutely yes)

When did your injury occur?   / ./
Before season, mid-season, or end season?

What is the nature of your injury?

What sport were you injured in?
How did it happen?

What specific goals do you have in sports?

Have they changed since the injury? (circle)
Yes / No   If yes, how?

How have you been feeling emotionally since the injury?

Please rank how these emotions describe how you are feeling because of the injury.
(12 = high, 0 = low)

...... Helpless   .... Tense
...... Bored   .... Depressed
...... Angry   .... Frustrated
...... Shocked   .... Discouraged
...... Frightened   .... Optimistic
...... In pain   .... Relieved
...... Other

If 0% is no recovery, what % recovery have you made to your pre-injury status? (circle)
0%   10%   20%   30%   40%   50%
      60%   70%   80%   90%   100%

When is your estimated date of return to sports?
   / /

Do you have fears about returning to sport? (circle)
Yes / No
If yes, what are they?

Are you a motivated person for exercise? (circle)
1   2   3   4   5   6   7   8   9   10
(not at all)   (extremely)

How well do you generally handle pain? (circle)
1   2   3   4   5
(not at all)   (somewhat)   (very well)

Are you encouraged in sports by your significant others? (circle)

Yes / No

Is this support: pressure   no support
                              just right?
Who exerts most pressure? (circle)
self   mother   father   coach   other

What are the major sources of stress in your life right now?

1   2

3   4

Were you under any recent stress (life changes) before the injury? (circle)   Yes / No
If yes, please describe

Do you have a strong family support system or close friends who know about your injury? (circle)

Yes / No   If yes, who are they? (ie. coach, friend, parents, teammates, other)

What do you think is the 'most important' thing necessary for your successful recovery?

Is the 'most important' thing something you have power over? (circle)

  1   2   3   4   5
(not at all)   (somewhat)   (very well)

How optimistic are you about fully recovering from your injury/surgery? (circle)

  1   2   3   4   5
(not at all)   (somewhat)   (very well)

What is your current rehabilitation program?
Exercises

        Times per week

Are you able to work out on exercise equipment or modalities? (circle)

Yes / No   If yes, please describe

Reprinted with permission from Adis Press. Smith, A. M., Scott, S. G., and Wiese, D. M. (1990). The Psychological effects of athletic injury: Coping. *Sports Medicine*, 9(6), p. 352–367.

Appendix B

The Profile of Mood States (POMS)

Below is an example of five of the 65 adjectives used on the POMS that describe the feelings people have. Circle ONE number under the answer that best describes HOW YOU HAVE BEEN FEELING DURING THE PAST WEEK, INCLUDING TODAY.

	Not at all	A little	Moderately	Quite a bit	Extremely
1. Friendly	0	1	2	3	4
2. Tense	0	1	2	3	4
3. Cheerful	0	1	2	3	4
4. Worthless	0	1	2	3	4
5. Shaky	0	1	2	3	4

Reprinted with permission. Write or call EDITS to obtain the tests, manual, and scoring key for this copyrighted measure. Order department: (619) 222-1666 or (800) 416-1666; Fax (619) 226-1666; E-mail: **edits@k-online.com;** Website: **www.edits.net**

Appendix C

Definitions Used in Sports Medicine Observation Code

<u>Active Rehabilitation.</u> The participant is in the process of receiving rehabilitation for an injury which was previously sustained. The objective of the rehabilitation is to restore the injured area to a good condition (e.g., icing the ankle, receiving ultrasound treatment).

<u>Initial Treatment.</u> The participant has sustained an injury within that day and is need of immediate first aid treatment (e.g., a basketball player has just turned over on his ankle during practice and is carried in for immediate treatment).

<u>Attending-Related.</u> The participant listens to what another person in the clinic is saying or watches what that person is doing. This person may be the athletic therapist, his coach, or another professional in the clinic. The attention being paid is directly related to the injury that was sustained.

<u>Attending-Unrelated.</u> The participant listens to what another person in the clinic is saying or watches what that person is doing. This person may be the athletic therapist, his coach, or another person in the clinic. The attention being paid is not directly related to his injury.

<u>Interaction-Related.</u> The participant interacts verbally with another person in the clinic. The discussion directly relates to the participant's injury. The participant may interact with the athletic therapist, his coach, or another person in the clinic.

<u>Interaction-Unrelated.</u> The participant interacts verbally with another person in the clinic. The discussion is not directly related to the participant's injury (e.g., topic of discussion may be the latest basketball game).

<u>Waiting</u>. The participant either waits for the doctor to assess the injury, for treatment, or waits to use equipment.

<u>Initial Diagnosis.</u> The physician/therapist attends to the participant and diagnoses the injury.

<u>Preventive Treatment.</u> The participant receives treatment that will prevent an injury from occurring (e.g., a varsity athlete has an ankle taped before practice).

<u>Maintenance.</u> The participant reports to the secretary to make an appointment, to fill out forms, or is preparing equipment for rehabilitation or

treatment (e.g., a person straps in his leg before using the Orthotron or places gel on the injured area before using ultrasound).

Non-Activity. The participant spends time in the clinic doing nothing (e.g., a person just stands or gazes and is not waiting or attending to the therapist or doctor).

Unrelated-Activity. The participant spends time on an activity which is not related to an injury and is not involved with any other person in the clinic (e.g., lying on a bench reading a book, walking from one room to another, or putting on a jacket to prepare to leave the clinic).

Exclusion. The participant leaves the clinic but returns within a short period of time (e.g., going to the washroom or for a drink of water).

Reprinted with permission from Dr. Jane Crossman. Crossman J. and Roch, J. (1991). An observational instrument for use in sports medicine clinics. *Canadian Journal of Physical Therapy*, April, 10–3.

Appendix D

Sport Inventory for Pain (SIP)

Below is a list of statements that describe the way athletes often feel about pain and it's influence on performance. Please take your time and read each statement carefully, so that we may find out how you feel toward pain. Then fill in one box to the right of each statement that describes your feelings at this time. Please answer honestly. There are no right or wrong answers.

	Strongly Disagree	Disagree	Neutral	Agree	Strongly Agree
1. I see pain as a challenge and don't let it bother me.	✿	✿	✿	✿	✿
2. I owe it to myself and those around me to perform even when my pain is bad.	✿	✿	✿	✿	✿
3. When in pain, I tell myself it doesn't hurt.	✿	✿	✿	✿	✿
4. When injured, I pray for the pain to stop.	✿	✿	✿	✿	✿
5. If I feel pain during a game, it=s probably a sign that I=m doing damage to my body.	✿	✿	✿	✿	✿
6. I have little or no trouble with my muscles twitching or jumping.	✿	✿	✿	✿	✿
7. At this point, I am more interested in returning to my sport than in trying to stop any pain.	✿	✿	✿	✿	✿
8. When in pain, I imagine that the pain is outside my body.	✿	✿	✿	✿	✿
9. When injured, I feel pain is terrible and that it=s never going to get better.	✿	✿	✿	✿	✿
10. When injured, I could perform as well as ever if my pain would go away.	✿	✿	✿	✿	✿
11. I do not worry about being injured.	✿	✿	✿	✿	✿
12. Pain is just a part of the game.	✿	✿	✿	✿	✿
13. When hurt, I play mental games with myself to keep my mind off the pain.	✿	✿	✿	✿	✿
14. When in pain, I worry all the time about whether it will end.	✿	✿	✿	✿	✿
15. When in pain, I have to be careful not to make it worse.	✿	✿	✿	✿	✿
16. I seldom or never have dizzy spells or headaches.	✿	✿	✿	✿	✿

17. When I am hurt, I just go on as if   ✿   ✿   ✿   ✿   ✿
    nothing happened.

18. When in pain, I replay in my mind   ✿   ✿   ✿   ✿   ✿
    pleasant performances from my past.

19. If in pain, I often feel I can=t stand   ✿   ✿   ✿   ✿   ✿
    it anymore.

20. The worse thing that could happen   ✿   ✿   ✿   ✿   ✿
    to me is to injure/reinjure myself.

21. I seldom notice minor injuries.   ✿   ✿   ✿   ✿   ✿

22. When injured, I tell myself to be   ✿   ✿   ✿   ✿   ✿
    tough and carry on despite the pain.

23. When hurt, I do anything to get   ✿   ✿   ✿   ✿   ✿
    my mind off the pain.

24. When hurt, I tell myself I can=t let   ✿   ✿   ✿   ✿   ✿
    the pain stand in the way of what
    I want to do.

25. No matter how bad the pain gets, I   ✿   ✿   ✿   ✿   ✿
    know I can handle it.

Scoring

Subscale	Items
Direct-Coping (COP)	1 + 2 + 7 +12 + 17 + 22 + 24 + 25
Cognitive (COG)	3 + 8 + 13 + 18 + 23
Catastrophizing (CAT)	4 + 9 + 14 + 19
Avoidance (AVD)	5 + 10 + 15 + 20
Body-Awareness (BOD)	6 + 11 + 16 + 21
Total Coping Response (TCR)	COP + COG B CAT

Appendix E

The Sports Injury Rehabilitation Beliefs Survey (SIRBS)

The words 'rehabilitation program' should be read to mean any advice that you are given in order to assist the rehabilitation of your injury.

Please respond to the following statements using the scale shown below:

Very Strongly Disagree	Strongly Disagree	Disagree	Neither Agree nor Disagree	Agree	Strongly Agree	Very Strongly Agree
1	2	3	4	5	6	7

1. My recovery from injury may be hindered if I do not complete the rehabilitation program.

       1   2   3   4   5   6   7

2. In order to prevent a recurrence of this injury, my rehabilitation program is essential.

       1   2   3   4   5   6   7

3. The way to prevent my injury from worsening will be to follow my rehabilitation program.

       1   2   3   4   5   6   7

4. A successful and lasting recovery may not be possible if I do not complete my rehabilitation program.

       1   2   3   4   5   6   7

5. I am making it more likely that I will be re-injured by not doing what my rehabilitation involves.

       1   2   3   4   5   6   7

6. The rehabilitation program designed for me will ensure my complete recovery from this injury.

       1   2   3   4   5   6   7

7. Completion of my rehabilitate program will guarantee that I recover from my injury.

       1   2   3   4   5   6   7

8. Following the advice that I have been given will have a very large impact upon how quickly I will recover from my injury.

       1   2   3   4   5   6   7

9. I have absolute faith in the effectiveness of my rehabilitation program.

       1   2   3   4   5   6   7

10. I am very capable of successfully completing all aspects of my rehabilitation program, even if it involves being less active or something that may be discomforting.

       1   2   3   4   5   6   7

11. I consider myself able to stick with my rehabilitation program even though it may include activities that I do not enjoy.

       1   2   3   4   5   6   7

12. I will have no serious difficulty in following the instructions of my rehabilitation program.

       1   2   3   4   5   6   7

13. I believe that I will stick to my rehabilitation program despite any difficulties that I may encounter.

| 1 | 2 | 3 | 4 | 5 | 6 | 7 |

14. Being fully recovered from injury is extremely important to me.

| 1 | 2 | 3 | 4 | 5 | 6 | 7 |

15. As far as injuries go, mine is serious.

| 1 | 2 | 3 | 4 | 5 | 6 | 7 |

16. I see this injury as a serious threat to my sport/exercise involvement.

| 1 | 2 | 3 | 4 | 5 | 6 | 7 |

17. I fear that this injury will affect my long-term sports involvement.

| 1 | 2 | 3 | 4 | 5 | 6 | 7 |

18. This injury is too serious to not follow medical advice.

| 1 | 2 | 3 | 4 | 5 | 6 | 7 |

19. Injuries like this are minor interruptions to my sport/exercise involvement.

| 1 | 2 | 3 | 4 | 5 | 6 | 7 |

Items 1–5 deal with susceptibility
Items 6–9 deal with treatment efficacy
Items 10–13 deal with self-efficacy
Item 14 deals with rehabilitation value
Items 15–19 deal with severity

Reprinted with permission from Dr. Adrian Taylor. Taylor, A. H., and May, S. (1996). Threat and coping appraisal as determinants of compliance to sports injury rehabilitation: An application of protection motivation theory. *Journal of Sports Sciences*, 14, 471–482.

Appendix F

Athletic Identity Measurement Scale (AIMS)

Please mark an **X** in the space that best reflects the extent to which you agree or disagree with each statement in relation to your own sports participation.

1. I consider myself an athlete.
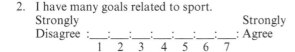
Strongly Disagree : : : : : : : Agree — 1 2 3 4 5 6 7

2. I have many goals related to sport.
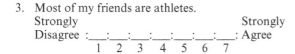
Strongly Disagree : : : : : : : Agree — 1 2 3 4 5 6 7

3. Most of my friends are athletes.
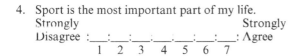
Strongly Disagree : : : : : : : Agree — 1 2 3 4 5 6 7

4. Sport is the most important part of my life.
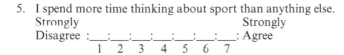
Strongly Disagree : : : : : : : Agree — 1 2 3 4 5 6 7

5. I spend more time thinking about sport than anything else.
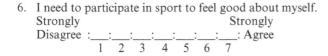
Strongly Disagree : : : : : : : Agree — 1 2 3 4 5 6 7

6. I need to participate in sport to feel good about myself.
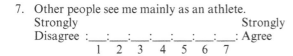
Strongly Disagree : : : : : : : Agree — 1 2 3 4 5 6 7

7. Other people see me mainly as an athlete.
Strongly Disagree : : : : : : : Agree — 1 2 3 4 5 6 7

8. I feel bad about myself when I do poorly in sport.
Strongly Disagree : : : : : : : Agree — 1 2 3 4 5 6 7

9. Sport is the only important thing in my life.
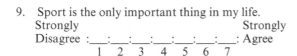
Strongly Disagree : : : : : : : Agree — 1 2 3 4 5 6 7

10.   I would be very depressed if I were injured and could not compete in sport.
Strongly   Strongly
Disagree :___:___:___:___:___:___:___: Agree
                 1   2   3   4   5   6   7

To score the AIMS, sum the scores of the ten items. The scores for each item range from 1 (strongly disagree) to 7 (strongly agree). Therefore, the higher your total score, the higher your athletic identity is.

SCORE	IDENTITY
49–70	High, exclusive
30–49	Moderate
7–30	Low

Reprinted with permission from Dr. Britt Brewer.

3   *The physician's viewpoint*

David F. Gerrard

Introduction

If really truthful, most physicians will acknowledge that their medical undergraduate years were grossly deficient in clinical sports medicine training and
even more bereft of any understanding for the emotional needs of the athlete
after the unexpected intrusion of injury or ill-health. The responses of the
athlete to injury have been widely observed and well described[1–3] and vary
from absolute frustration to depression and uncontrollable anger.[4] Some
have even compared an athlete's reaction to injury to a process of grieving a
significant personal loss.

The aim of this chapter is to describe the role of the physician by detail-
ing the mechanism of sports injury, considering the profile of the 'at-risk'
athlete, proposing a role for the physician during rehabilitation, and discussing the assessment of the athlete before a safe return to sport is advisable.

No matter how well prepared an athlete might be in the physical sense, the
intervention of injury or ill-health prior to competition will limit performance and will limit the earning potential of the professional athlete. Some
illnesses may be unavoidable, but contemporary athletes are expected to
assume a greater degree of responsibility for their personal fitness and health.
Injury interferes with training, impedes performance, can influence team
selection, and ultimately impacts upon income. Athletes have become more
knowledgeable about injury prevention, sports first aid, and rehabilitation
principles, banned and permitted drugs, and aspects of nutrition.
Professional sport has also spawned an expansion of support staff to include
specialist sports physicians, orthopaedic surgeons, psychologists, physiotherapists, fitness advisors, massage therapists, nutritionists, strength trainers,
and other health-related professionals.

High-performance sport injury or ill health assume no less importance to
the recreational athlete, as to the high-performance athlete.[6] Time lost from
habituated exercise is frustrating to those for whom regular physical activity
is a significant feature in their life. Their rights to appropriate clinical attention are no less deserving. Therefore, in this chapter, no distinction will inten-

tionally be made between the high-performance athlete and the regular-exercise enthusiast. These two groups share common physical and emotional responses and it would be unwise of any physician to apply different management principles. Given the range of support services available to high-profiled athletes, there will likely be an accelerated mechanism of primary care and referral compared to the average person. Notwithstanding this fact, the pathology of, for example, a ruptured tendoachilles in a recreational skier is no different to that occurring in a professional footballer. The pathophysiology is no different, rehabilitation principles are similar, and arguably the only difference is the expectant level of physical demand when the athlete returns to the 'field of play'.

Classifying injury in sport

Sport injury has frequently been described as an occupational hazard; particularly in high-velocity, impact sports. There have been significant changes to the management of the injured player, and these advances owe their genesis to professional sport where greater resources have allowed clinical techniques to become more refined and rehabilitation techniques to improve. Athletes, in whom financial investments are huge, are assessed with urgency and transferred rapidly for appropriate specialized care. Indirectly, a classification of injury has emerged that has benefited all injured athletes, professional and non-professional alike.

This classification takes into account the mechanism of the injury and highlights a simple process of history-taking that is the foundation of diagnosis taught to medical students in their early clinical careers. Primary or field assessment, sports first aid, and critical diagnostic clues are obtained from such a thorough history.

The most serious category of injury results from external forces that typify 'contact' sport. Usually there is a collision with a stationary object or impact between two bodies frequently moving in opposite directions. In such cases, fractured limbs, dislocated joints, trauma to internal organs, ruptured ligaments, head and neck injuries, or concussion are common and may carry serious consequences. Sports such as football, skiing, horse-riding, martial arts, and motor racing are commonly implicated in this type of injury. The critical features of these sports are high velocity and impact. Prompt medical intervention is essential, and at times life-saving. The athlete may be concussed or seriously immobilized. Effective injury management begins on the field of play where the injured athlete must be handled with skill and care. Apart from the need for expert primary assessment and support, there is frequently a demand for special investigations including radiographs, computed tomography (CT) scanning, or magnetic resonance imaging (MRI). Examples of such injuries include:

- a fracture dislocation of the cervical spine of a rugby player who is unexpectedly caught in the middle of a collapsing scrum;

- a severe, closed head injury in an equestrian eventer who falls from his/her horse at a difficult cross-country jump;

- a fractured ankle in an artistic gymnast who lands awkwardly from a difficult beam dismount;

- a ruptured anterior cruciate ligament in the knee of a downhill ski racer who crashes a difficult slalom gate at high speed.

A definable traumatic incident is always a feature of the history and, until proven otherwise, one must assume that a serious musculoskeletal, or internal injury, has occurred. Almost without exception, these athletes are unable to continue and are literally 'stretchered off' for medical attention.

The other category of injury represents a spectrum of trauma resulting from repetitive forces generated by ballistic, bouncing, weight-bearing activities like jogging. These forces are responsible for overused or torn muscles, inflamed tendons, strained ligaments, and stress reactions in bone. Although such injuries pose less serious clinic challenges and are less dramatic in their presentation, they are no less troublesome to the enthusiastic athlete. These are the typical overuse injuries, and they represent the largest group of injuries seen in every sports medicine clinic. Examples include:

- a stress fracture in the shin of the 'social' jogger through failing to wear road shoes appropriate to his or her foot biomechanics;

- chronic pain in the dominant shoulder of the waterpolo player as a consequence of an undisclosed impingement syndrome aggravated by repetitive throwing;

- an overuse tendinitis in the wrist of the tennis player, associated with incorrect technique and racquet size;

- a traction injury of the quadriceps attachment in the knee of the young soccer player, through excessive kicking drills.

The common feature of these injuries is that there is commonly no single, identifiable event to which a specific injury may be attributed. The symptoms are frequently longstanding, commonly aggravated by exercise, and inevitably improved by rest.

At-risk athletes

Several epidemiological studies have identified characteristics that appear common to at-risk or 'injury-prone' athletes.[5,7–9] The New Zealand Rugby Injury and Performance Project (RIPP) studied a cohort of 356 rugby union players during a complete season of competition.[10] Rugby football is the national sport of New Zealand played by over 100,000 participants. In epidemiological terms it represents the archetypal contact sport and has the highest rate of injury of all major sports in New Zealand. Although a traditional male bastion, rugby in New Zealand is now played widely by women and the national women's team (the Black Ferns) is the current World champion. A multidisciplinary group, using a prospective, cohort, study design sought to establish past injury experience, identify the influence of previous injury, monitor the use of safety equipment, and determine the significance of medical advice to injured rugby players.[11] Baseline data obtained from questionnaires were used to establish a positive relationship between past injury experience and the prediction of injury during the season. A disturbingly large number of players (39%) continued to play rugby despite medical advice to the contrary and the use of prophylactic ankle strapping, head pro-

INJURY
The result of an acute or chronic process
ACUTE MANAGEMENT
Primary assessment and the initiation of sports first aid (RICE)
CLINICAL EXAMINATION
An accurate history of the injury and psychological impact
INVESTIGATIONS
To exclude or confirm clinical suspicions
DIAGNOSIS
Obtained from the synthesis of history, examination and investigations
TREATMENT PLAN
Collaboration with colleagues in physical, psychological and biomechanical disciplines
REHABILITATION
The restoration of normal structure, function, confidence and esteem
ASSESSMENT OF FITNESS
A coordinated process to ensure a safe return to previous activity

Fig. 3.1   A model for managing injury in sport.

tection, and body padding were typically linked to chronic injury. Return to play before full rehabilitation had been achieved was another disturbing pattern to emerge. These findings represented the attitudes of a cohort of amateur rugby players whose playing careers were not influenced by professional management or franchises. Nevertheless, a rather cavalier attitude towards injury, the inappropriate use of 'pain killers' and a disregard for rehabilitation principles was evident and common to other reports of intercollegiate athletes.[7] For the most part, injured players in this study interpreted medical advice as being at the most conservative end of the therapeutic spectrum and few, if any, received any qualified psychological support.

Key physical and psychological characteristics of the 'at-risk' athlete are often helpful in alerting team support personnel to the potential for non-compliance with respect to rehabilitation.[5] Stress factors may arise as a direct consequence of sport participation, or may be related to personal environmental influences such as the level of competition, position on the team, and individual leadership responsibilities.[7]

The physician's role in rehabilitation

Effective rehabilitation represents a partnership between a number of healthcare practitioners, with the injured athlete their common focus.[6] Central to this concept is the establishment of an accurate diagnosis that is the prime responsibility of the attending physician, with whom the total well-being of the athlete ought to reside. To establish a diagnosis one must first obtain an accurate history, undertake a comprehensive physical examination, and then initiate appropriate investigations to either eliminate or confirm clinical suspicions. The physician who cares for athletes must be trained in the practical knowledge of a number of disciplines. An understanding of the principles of physical therapy, biomechanics, psychology, exercise prescription, and nutrition must be within the capabilities of all sports physicians. Only then can they be capable of seeking the assistance of the appropriate colleague or rehabilitative agency.

By definition, rehabilitation infers the restoration of normal structure and function. To facilitate this, the physician requires the full confidence of the injured athlete. This begins with the early application of measures to modulate the overwhelming effect of the acute inflammatory response. This is best achieved through the simple first-aid measures of rest, ice, compression, and elevation, popularized by the well-known acronym RICE. The use of anti-inflammatory, analgesic medication may also be appropriate at this stage, but must only be administered through legitimate medical channels and not at the whim of a well-meaning team-mate or trainer. After undertaking investigations to confirm an accurate diagnosis it is critical for the physician to communicate with three individual groups of people.

First, and of greatest importance, is the athlete, to whom a simple, clear and honest explanation is mandatory. This must include an outline of the proposed treatment plan, a likely prognosis, and, most importantly, a realistic time-frame for recovery. Experience confirms that those patients who have a good knowledge of their clinical problem achieve the best results.[4] These athletes have been described as having willingness to '...learn and listen, and are motivated and determined.'[12] A good rapport between physician and patient engenders this confidence. Athlete compliance, critical for a satisfactory rehabilitation outcome, is directly related to this relationship. A competent clinician should always be prepared to discuss second opinions and entertain alternative therapies provided they have a sound basis, are ethically and legally acceptable, and cause the athlete no ill-effect. Similarly, the physician should argue against 'quick fix' remedies to satisfy a rapid and, frequently temporary, return to activity. In some instances this argument has its genesis in the indirect pressure applied by the coach, administration, or even team sponsors. The inappropriate use of analgesic (painkilling) medication is a common example frequently not in the best long-term interests of the athlete, but which satisfies the immediate demand of coach, team, and sponsor. An athlete may well feel a divided loyalty in these instances, and the independence of the physician can shift the onus of responsibility from the athlete. The ethical, contractual, and legal obligations of all members of the medical support staff must be clearly defined and understood before assuming any professional responsibility for a team.[13] The health of the athlete must remain paramount. The physician can facilitate this entire process by providing the athlete with a clear and understandable explanation of the diagnosis, prognosis, and rehabilitation plan.

Another example of contemporary conflict in sports medicine is the intrusion of performance-enhancing drugs. Team physicians may gain knowledge of the illicit use of drugs by athletes through the confidentiality of the consultation room. The dilemma of how to deal with such information rests with the individual physician who must account for ethical and moral obligations and the overriding well-being of the patient.[13]

The next group with whom consultation is important is the coaching staff who may have preconceived and totally unrealistic expectations of the rehabilitative process. They might also express their own anecdotal, unscientific preference for treatment. However, with the full permission of the athlete, it is important to discuss the nature of the injury and prognosis with the coach who is then more likely to support and respect the decision of the physician. Once again this discussion should to be conducted with honesty, frankness, and a willingness to consider all therapeutic options. The collective coaching staff also deserves to be regularly updated on the injured athlete's progress and this demands a clear line of communication with the athlete's full consent. In the case of individual athletes, particularly young ones, there is often an ominous influence of the overbearing, anxious parent. This is more common in sports like swimming, gymnastics, and dance and those activities that encourage early competition such as little-league baseball. There is a strong argument that young athletes should be acquiring a wide range of useful skills rather than learning to become intensely competitive. While the preadolescent athlete is at risk of a number of musculoskeletal problems, less well recognized is the psychological and emotional trauma that they frequently suffer at the hands of unsparing parents and clamorous coaches.[14] Many clinicians will be aware that the demands of parents are often more significant than those of the coach. As a physician, I have found that tact and consistency are positive measures helpful in dealing with the unrealistic expectations of the overbearing parent. The temptation to provide short-term, 'patch up' assistance to young athletes is not acting in accordance with a professional approach to their long-term health and well-being.

Third, and critical to the success of any rehabilitative process, is the relationship between physician and other healthcare professionals. There is no rigid sequence of communication or collaboration because every injury scenario is unique. Frequently, there may be financial limitations that govern the extent of ancillary rehabilitative services affordable by the 'non-professional', less-insured athlete.

Some athletes are fiercely independent and self-reliant. They are sufficiently motivated to proceed with their own rehabilitation programme with the minimum of external input. Others are outrageously dependent upon as many physical and emotional support services that can be mustered. 'Training room dependence' has been recognized by many researchers.[4] Between these two extremes of dependency, clinicians will agree that there lies an 'average' athlete whose response to injury is displayed by the behavioural traits of '...adjustment and appropriate emotion'.[4] The assessment and management of these individuals becomes the clinical responsibility of the sport psychologist in whom the wise sports physician will invest great faith. The wisdom associated with such referrals develops from the physician's experience and understanding of the capabilities of the individual psychologist. From the physical perspective, the rehabilitative regime requires active input from physiotherapists who utilize the modalities of electrotherapy and early, active mobilization so critical to successful rehabilitation. Emotional influences are not so quantifiable, and the athlete's psychological welfare is frequently overlooked both at the time of injury and also when some element of 'fitness testing' becomes timely. Measures of psychological influence are well reported and a useful example is the Emotional Responses of Athletes to Injury Questionnaire described in the previous chapter.[15]

Return to play

Tradition has dictated that the return of any athlete to sport is pre-empted by some measure of preparedness, that has rather euphemistically become known as a 'fitness test'. This typically includes quantitative measures of strength, speed, endurance, proprioceptive ability, or muscle bulk. Frequently omitted is some determination of psychological status. A return of confidence, improved self-esteem, and other indicators of intrinsic recovery are much less quantifiable. It is therefore clear that any decision about returning to play should be made on the basis of collaboration between athlete, physician, sport psychologist, and coach (or significant other). In the case of a healing fracture, the endpoint may be radiologically definable and the self-limiting nature of the injury makes the decision quite simple. Less defined are injuries that have arisen from a chronic, repetitive, overuse mechanism. Unless the rehabilitative process has included some dramatic preventive strategy, there can be no guarantee that the problem will not recur. Quite clearly, in these situations, the athlete has less confidence.[2]

The physician may report clinical recovery and the coach may record acceptable measures of physical 'fitness', but these two opinions may not concur with the athlete's personal perception of his/her status. In such a case, return to play would be unwise and recognition of the athlete's judgement is critical. Similarly, where the athlete's perception of preparedness is in advance of medical and coaching advice, the dangers of a premature return to sport must all be recognized. Either way, the use of psychological counselling is both appropriate and advisable. Return to play should only occur when all the pieces of the rehabilitative puzzle come together. Pressure from external sources, such as sponsors and fans, must be set aside and regarded as secondary to the well-being of the athlete. There are numerous anecdotal tales of athletes returning prematurely for the 'critical' game, players participating under the influence of painkilling injections, and graphic descriptions of heroic efforts by debilitated performers. Despite these memorable stories, it remains for us all to observe respect for the athlete's overall welfare. From the wider perspective, there is plenty of life after sport and the younger the athlete, the more important the shared, professional responsibility to ensure that these are quality years.

The following case studies provide typical scenarios that illustrate how psychological influences may distract the injured athlete from the long-term goals of complete recovery. In the first, a talented young rugby player is pressured to return to play prematurely, but ultimately realizes that his health is suffering and that long-term goals really are worth the wait. The second highlights the inappropriate pressures applied to a gymnast by her coach and parents who disregard her physical and emotional safety to satisfy their personal Olympic aspirations.

Case study 1

An 18-year-old, university student, rugby player suffered multiple concussions during a normal club season. This player was widely regarded as having the potential to play first grade rugby and possibly even achieve international status. His injury profile was documented by the University Student Health Service where he was under the care of a sports physician. After one significant concussion this player disregarded a mandatory 3-week period away from contact sport to play in an important representative trial from which he was named for junior provincial honours. He then reported recurring headaches and mild visual disturbance to his physician. These were fully investigated and even in the absence of any abnormalities on CT scanning and MRI, he was advised to withdraw from all contact sport for the remainder of the season. Disregarding considerable pressure from his coaches, the player complied with the advice of his physician. He volunteered to end the season prematurely and decided to take time off in the following season when his symptoms showed no signs of remission. During this time he resisted the continued pressure from coaches and team-mates and chose to assist with the coaching and administration of his former team. The following year, free from any significant symptoms and declared medically fit this player returned to a career in professional rugby that has taken him to the highest international levels. He is considered by many to be the best rugby player in his position in the world.

Case study 2

A 14-year-old artistic gymnast suffered chronic left shin pain in the lead up to the Olympic trials. This was diagnosed initially as 'shin splints' and treated conservatively. As the current national champion, her selection seemed a foregone conclusion. However, the symptoms persisted and limited her ability to train. In fact, further investigations revealed that she had developed a stress reaction in her tibial shaft and, although able to continue training, the postexercise symptoms were so severe that she began to use regular painkilling medication. Increasing pressure from coach and parents encouraged an urgency to tolerate discomfort to fulfil a lifelong Olympic dream. Medical advice, strongly counter to this opinion, was disregarded. Despite a confidential 'cry for help' to the sports physician, the personal feelings of this young gymnast were essentially ignored. She lost confidence in many of her basic routines and her overall performance fell well below par. The coach then enlisted the aid of a sports psychologist to restore her confidence and retrieve some lost form. One week later during a difficult dismount from the uneven bars she landed heavily and fractured her left tibia at the site of the previous stress reaction. Urgent orthopaedic intervention was necessary and her Olympic aspirations were shattered. Sadly this talented athlete has never wished to compete again.

Conclusions

There is always a risk of injury associated with any form of physical endeavour. However, this risk is reduced when common-sense principles are adhered to and athletes are well prepared, willing to abide by the rules, and heed signs of physical or emotional malfunction. External pressures from a number of significant others may influence athletes to disregard important signals and play through pain. Support from a range of healthcare professionals is essential for athletes to identify their problem and obtain appropriate therapy. Central to this is the sports physician with whom athletes must have rapport and in whom there must be absolute trust.

The role of the physician in the rehabilitative process is fivefold, and these important functions are summarized as follows:

(1) to develop the confidence of the injured athlete through an open and honest relationship;

(2) to expedite a speedy and accurate diagnosis;

(3) to facilitate the collaboration of expertise to obtain the best rehabilitative outcome that provides overall health and welfare;

(4) to maintain regular dialogue with coach, parents, and significant others with the knowledge and consent of the athlete; and

(5) to ensure that the return to sport is timely for the athlete and takes account of appropriate preventive strategies.

While the prophets of doom continue to count the public cost of sport-related injury, it may be argued that an active population is healthier, happier, and in the long run more productive.

References

1. Evans L. and Hardy, L. (1995). Sport injury and grief responses: A review. *Journal of Sport and Exercise Psychology,* **17**, 227–45.
2. Petrie, G. (1993). Injury from the athlete's point of view. In *Psychology of sport injury* (ed. J. Heil), pp. 17–23. Human Kinetics, Champaign, IL.
3. Quackenbush, N. and Crossman, J. (1994). Injured athletes: A study of emotional responses. *Journal of Sports Behaviour,* **17**, 178–87.
4. Crossman, J. (1997). Psychological rehabilitation from sports injuries. *Sports Medicine,* **23**, 333–9.
5. Grove, J. R. and Gordon, A. M. D. (1995). The psychological aspects of injury in sport. In *Science and medicine in sport* (2nd edn) (ed. J. Bloomfield, P. A. Fricker, and K. D. Fitch), pp. 194–205. Blackwell Scientific, Carlton, Victoria, Australia.
6. Steadman, J. R. (1993). A physician's approach to the psychology of injury. In *Psychology of sport injury* (ed. J. Heil), pp. 25–31. Human Kinetics, Champaign, IL.
7. Sachs, M. L., Sitier, M. R., and Schwille, G. (1993). Assessing and monitoring injuries in inter-collegiate athletes: A counseling/prediction model. In *Psychological bases of sport injuries* (ed. D. Pargman), pp. 71–84. Fitness Information Technology, Morgantown, WV.

8. Garraway, M. and MacLeod, D. (1995). Epidemiology of rugby football injuries. *Lancet,* **345**, 1485–7.

9. Hughes D. C. and Fricker, P. A. (1994). A prospective survey of injuries to first-grade rugby union players. *Clinical Journal of Sport Medicine,* **4**, 249–56.

10. Waller, A. E., Feehan, M., Marshall, S. M., and Chalmers, D. J. (1994). The New Zealand rugby injury and performance project: 1. Design and methodology of a prospective follow-up study. *British Journal of Sports Medicine,* **28**, 223–8.

11. Gerrard, D. F., Waller, A. E., and Bird, Y. N. (1994). The New Zealand rugby injury and performance project: II. Previous injury experience of a rugby-playing cohort. *British Journal of Sports Medicine,* **28**, 229–33.

12. Wiese, D. M., Weiss, M. R., and Yukelson, D. P. (1991). Sport psychology in the training room: A survey of athletic trainers. *The Sport Psychologist,* **5**, 15–24.

13. Makarowski, L. M. and Rickell, J. G. (1993). Ethical and legal issues for sport professionals counseling injured athletes. In *Psychological bases of sport injuries* (ed. D. Pargman), pp. 45–65. Fitness Information Technology, Morgantown, WV.

14. Gerrard, D. F. (2000). The dilemma of the young athlete. *New Ethicals,* **3**, 1.

15. Smith, A. M. (1996). Psychological impact of injuries in athletes. *Sports Medicine,* **22**, 391–405.

4 *The role of the physiotherapist and sport therapist*

Sandy Gordon, Margaret Potter, and Peter Hamer

Introduction

This chapter has three objectives: first, to provide a brief overview of research that supports the use of sport psychology principles and mental skills techniques as part of the rehabilitation process for injured athletes; second, to outline a periodization approach for the application of mental skills techniques related to the pathology and repair phases of rehabilitation; and third, to illustrate with three case studies how mental skills training can be implemented within guidelines for best practice.

Overview of research: what rehabilitation professionals have reported

It is likely that any physical impairment which prohibits physical activity in an athlete, whether temporary or permanent, will be cognitively, emotionally, and behaviorally challenging.[1] In addition to the sudden cessation of various positive experiences associated with participation in sport, athletes have to deal with physical losses (e.g. endurance, agility, speed, power) and skill losses (e.g. form, ability), and significant changes in identity (e.g. self-concept, belief system, social and perhaps occupational functioning).[2,3] While the most common experience of symbolic loss relates to athletic identity, other forms of loss are also possible, such as mobility, independence, sense of control, status, confidence, virility, daily routine, social ties, and income opportunities or financial rewards.[3,4]

The psychological sequelae of sport injuries can result in distress, which, in injured athletes, can manifest itself in several ways: non-acceptance of the injury; denial of the seriousness or extent of the injury; displays of depression, anger, apprehension, or anxiety; failure to take responsibility for personal rehabilitation; non-adherence to a rehabilitation program; missing appointments; overdoing rehabilitation; non-cooperation with rehabilitation strategies; bargaining with rehabilitation professionals over treatment or the time out of competition; frequent negative statements about the injury and rehabilitation; reduced effort, poor attention, and intensity in rehabilitation; unconfirmable reports of pain; inappropriate behavior outside rehabilitation, e.g. using the injured area; inappropriate emotions; and emotional swings.[5–7]

In addition to the above manifestations of distress, several surveys of sport physiotherapists,[5,8] physical therapists,[9] sport/athletic trainers,[8–10] and sport physicians[11] have revealed that the most frequent and significant emotions and behaviors associated with unsuccessful treatment in athletes include: fear and anxiety; anger and frustration; lack of understanding of the injury and recovery process; and wanting to return to competition before full recovery. Similar findings are also reported from research on athletes' experiences with injury and recovery[12–16] and highlight both the strong emotional and behavioral consequences of sport injury and the significant role psychology plays in the overall management of injured athletes.

Sport-injury rehabilitation professionals have also reported that certain psychological interventions and strategies are often required to overcome the emotions and behaviors experienced by injured athletes. If understood and used properly, these strategies are valuable tools in the facilitation of effective rehabilitation. Specifically, sport physiotherapists and sport/athletic trainers believe the following mental skills are important and desirable components of their education: goal setting and motivation techniques; communication and counseling skills; arousal control and anxiety management; confidence and assertiveness training; concentration and attentional control; cognitive restructuring (controlling thought processes); reduction of depression; pain management; relaxation; imagery or visualization; and the provision of social support.[8,10,17,18] It is interesting that these findings are consistent with the research that has focused on identifying strategies that athletes can employ to maintain motivation and persistence, solve problems, and cope more effectively during the healing process.[12,19–23]

Mental skills training: which skills and when?

The use of mental skills training during rehabilitation from sport injury has been employed by a number of researchers and is advocated to assist recovery.[19,24–29] In particular, the techniques of collaborative goal-setting, imagery, relaxation training, positive self-talk, and effective communication skills to enhance the interaction between the injured athlete and sports medicine personnel have been suggested.[3,25–27,29–31] These techniques can be applied during rehabilitation to help athletes cope with pain and anxiety, deal with negative and irrational thinking, and to assist with motivation and compliance.

Table 4.1   Periodized mental skills training during sport injury rehabilitation

Phase	Likely 'mental demands' on an injured athlete	Foundation skills	Techniques
1. Immediate postinjury (inflammatory reaction)	Behaviors indicative of a grief-like response High-level anxiety Problems coping with pain Negative attitude to injury and life Lack of social support	Counselling regarding the grief-response Anxiety management Relaxation training Cognitive restructuring Social support	Communication skills-explain injury and proposed treatment. Discover what the injury means to the individual. Answer athlete's questions Arousal control/anxiety management Autogenic training Thought-stopping and positive self-talk Provide emotional and informational and/or tangible support
2. Early to progressive rehabilitation (Tissue regeneration and repair)	Non-compliance Failure to take responsibility Dysfunctional attitude Lack of understanding of the healing process Lack of focus or goals Lack of motivation Lack of self-confidence and self-worth	Counseling Cognitive restructuring Imagery Self-awareness/self-regulation Building confidence	Communication skills—clarify the therapist's expectations of the athlete. Distinguish pain of healing from pain signaling further injury. Prepare athlete for plateaus and possible setbacks. Answer the athlete's questions Body rehearsal of the healing process Collaborative goal-setting (task-focused) Confidence/assertiveness training
3. Advanced rehabilitation (Tissue maturation)	A continuation of phase 2	Potentially any of the foundation skills	Communication skills—encouragement and challenge Goal-setting (motivational) Imagery (mastery rehearsal for return to sport) Concentration/attention control

Providing therapists with a 'periodized plan', as illustrated in Table 4.1, may make it easier for them to both identify and implement mental skills-training techniques in conjunction with the physical rehabilitation plan. To facilitate the use of this framework, the techniques that are appropriate within each phase are discussed below. The utilization of mental skills techniques will be dependent on the knowledge and skills of the therapist and assessed 'individual needs', and any of the techniques may be applicable at any stage.

Communication skills

Communication (verbal, non-verbal, and written) provides the essence of the relationship between the therapist and the injured athlete.

Phase 1: immediate postinjury

It is important to create a comfortable environment and for the therapist to be aware of verbal and non-verbal behavior from the outset.[32] Part of the initial rapport building process will involve the therapist attempting to attain an understanding of what the injury means to the athlete.[3] By doing so, the injured athlete is likely to feel understood and that they can trust the therapist enough to share their concerns. The initial treatment session should include spending time to educate the athlete about the injury, proposed treatment, and expectations for recovery. This may include the use of aids such as anatomical models, diagrams, video and computer graphics, and the provision of written information for the injured athlete. Therapists should be receptive to questions from the injured athlete. If there is insufficient time to answer all questions, or not enough information is available for a response, a follow-up session should be planned for a subsequent visit. Alternatively, it may be necessary for therapists to liaise with other healthcare professionals to obtain feedback or to refer the injured athlete onwards.

Phase 2: early to progressive rehabilitation

As rehabilitation progresses, much of the communication between the injured athlete and therapist will focus on goal-setting and clarification of the athlete's questions and concerns. A number of issues may be raised, including pain levels, client versus therapist expectations during rehabilitation, appropriate modification to activities, frustration with the rehabilitation process, motivation and compliance. What should the athlete expect as they start to become more mobile? Can the therapist assist the athlete to distinguish between pain associated with healing and pain that may signal further injury? The therapist must be prepared for such questions or be willing to seek answers on behalf of the injured athlete. In addition, at this stage it is sensible to prepare the athlete for potential setbacks and plateaus in the rehabilitation process. While they may not encounter any obstacles in their progress, it is advisable to be proactive since an unexpected setback could adversely affect the athlete's motivation and compliance.

Phase 3: advanced rehabilitation

During the later stages of rehabilitation, the therapist should be aware of the potential for the athlete's motivation to wane. The focus of communication will be to challenge athletes while encouraging their efforts and reinforcing collaborative goal-setting strategies.

Collaborative goal-setting

Once an injury has occurred it is essential to devise an appropriate management plan to provide a rehabilitation framework. The importance of the injured athlete's active participation in this process has been emphasized by a number of researchers.[26,30,33,34]

Phase 1: immediate postinjury

As part of the assessment, diagnosis, and initial management of the injury, the therapist must spend time educating the athlete on what to expect and the proposed treatment plan. Collaborative goal-setting should be integral to the initial management, including the process of obtaining a complete diagnosis, e.g. referral for other medical investigations. Once the diagnosis is clear, the therapist and injured athlete should discuss and set goals for the roles each will play in the rehabilitation process. There needs to be an exchange of views

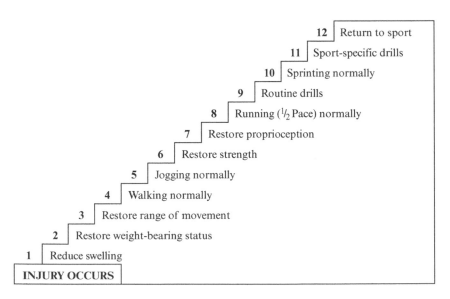

Fig. 4.1   An example of a rehabilitation goal-setting staircase for treating an ankle sprain. (Adapted with permission from ref. 26.)

so that the injured athlete is able to share his or her thoughts and feelings with the physiotherapist.[35] At this stage, it is critical that the injured athlete is given as much information as possible and made aware of what will be involved during the physical rehabilitation process. A rehabilitation staircase, as illustrated in Fig. 4.1, is often useful to convey the various stages of recovery to the injured athlete. At the first or second treatment session, a copy can be made for the athlete to take away with them. This will help to put the injury and their position in the rehabilitation process in perspective and may prompt them to ask questions and take an active role.

Phase 2: early to progressive rehabilitation

As physical rehabilitation progresses, the injured athlete will become more involved in undertaking the appropriate exercises. Collaborative goals should be set at each treatment session to help both the injured athlete and therapist to focus on each step in the rehabilitation process. Short-term (e.g. weekly), medium term (e.g. monthly), and long-term (e.g. 6–12 month) goals will also need to be established depending on the severity of injury and likely length of rehabilitation. These goals may be related to the physical or mental aspects of rehabilitation. Completion of an appropriately designed rehabilitation goals sheet, as illustrated in Table 4.2, will ensure that goals set are 'SMARTER', i.e. specific, measurable, acceptable, realistic, time-based, evaluated, and recorded. (For further information refer to Chapter 6.)

Table 4.2   SMARTER rehabilitation goals sheet

Specific	GOAL: Date set:
Measurable	How can I measure improvement? Examples: Reduction in pain, swelling, and full range of movement—feedback from the therapist. Ability to complete specific drills set up by the therapist.
Acceptable	What do I have to do? Examples: Do some individual sessions with the therapist. Do my rehabilitation exercises.
Realistic	How am I going to do this? Example: Attend the rehabilitation clinic twice/week.
Time-based	When will I achieve this goal? Example: 1 week, 1 month, etc.
Evaluated	How will I know I have achieved it? Example: Ability to successfully complete my rehabilitation program goals set in conjunction with my therapist.
Recorded	Monitor and record Write it down. 'Ink it, don't just think it!'

Phase 3: advanced rehabilitation

Appropriate goal-setting is essential during the later stages of recovery, when motivation may be a problem, particularly in long-term rehabilitation. It can provide motivation and commitment, direct the injured athlete's attention to controllable factors, and help to build confidence.[31,35-37]

Anxiety management

Anxiety often accompanies injury and may manifest itself in various emotional responses of the injured athlete. Research has reported frustration, depression, and boredom among injured sports people who demonstrated more negative mood postinjury when compared with normative data.[38] These behaviors may be detrimental to effective rehabilitation.

Phase 1: immediate postinjury

The need to inform the injured athletes about what to expect is important for reducing their uncertainty, anxiety, and pain[39] and information should include education regarding the diagnosis and treatment plan. Additionally, it will help if the therapist can allay the athletes' fears by encouraging them to ask questions and being able to provide detailed, appropriate explanations at a suitable level of understanding for the particular athlete. This information exchange will empower the athletes helping them take some control in the rehabilitation process through collaborative goal-setting with the therapist.

Phase 2: early to progressive rehabilitation

If the athlete is making the expected progress in rehabilitation, it is unlikely that high anxiety will be a significant feature during this phase. However, if a setback is encountered, anxiety may return as the athlete is forced to deal with unexpected events. During this time, it is important that the therapist re-evaluate the treatment plan with the athlete so that goals are modified as necessary. In addition, the therapist needs to be available to answer the inevitable questions that are likely to arise from the athlete such as: 'Why has this setback occurred?' 'Am I ever going to get better?'

Phase 3: advanced rehabilitation

Generally at this stage, anxiety related to the occurrence of the injury is less pronounced. However, the injured athlete may experience anxiety related to returning to sport. If this is the case, appropriate strategies that could be useful include relaxation training,[40] goal-setting, and imagery focused on mastery rehearsal for a successful return to sport.

Relaxation training

Physiological changes indicating an improvement in relaxation, such as decreases in heart rate, respiration rate, and blood pressure, have been demonstrated with relaxation training.[40] Relaxation training is reported to assist an injured athlete to cope with pain[39,41,42] and affect the sympathetic nervous system to aid healing.[34,43]

Phase 1: immediate postinjury

Autogenic relaxation is a very useful technique to implement during this rehabilitation phase, as it has the potential to moderate the inflammatory reaction that occurs immediately postinjury.[34,43] This form of relaxation training systematically focuses the athlete's attention on relaxing individual body parts by inducing the sensation of warmth and heaviness in each area. Furthermore, the injured athlete can use this technique to 'visualize' the healing process.

Phase 2: early to progressive rehabilitation

Building on techniques introduced immediately postinjury, relaxation training can assist with both pain control and anxiety management and be further extended to assist with enhancing concentration, self-confidence, and self-control.[40]

Phase 3: Advanced rehabilitation

At this stage, relaxation training is unlikely to be a major component in the rehabilitation program. However, once taught it can be utilized by the injured athlete as a coping strategy for assisting with return-to-sport goals and dealing with other avenues of life, e.g. work stress or relationship problems. (For further information about relaxation training refer to Chapter 7.)

Cognitive strategies

Research into faulty or self-defeating inner dialogues reveals that evaluations, thoughts, feelings, and self-talk prior to, during, and following injury and rehabilitation are important determinants of subsequent behavior. It is common for injured athletes to have negative and irrational thoughts following a sport-injury,[3,16] for instance: 'this is hopeless, most athletes never recover from this injury'; 'this treatment lark is a waste of time—what do they (doctors and therapists) know?' Positive self-talk strategies can counteract dysfunctional thoughts by increasing an athlete's awareness and sensitivity to faulty thinking.

Phase 1: immediate postinjury

The introduction of a technique such as 'thought-stopping', to make the athlete aware of their thinking and to give them a strategy to change it, may be very beneficial. Thought-stoppage involves the athlete identifying the unwanted 'negative thought(s)' and then, using a trigger such as the word 'stop', to interrupt that thought. The trigger may be verbal or non-verbal, but it must consistently be used by the athlete to eliminate undesirable thoughts.

Phase 2: early to progressive rehabilitation

Once the injured athlete has mastered thought-stoppage it can be progressed to changing negative thoughts to positive statements. This involves recognizing the negative thought(s), using a trigger to eliminate further negative thinking, and then replacing it with a positive statement. The negative thought for the injured athlete may be 'My leg is weak, I can't do anything!' As soon as this thought comes to mind the athlete says 'stop' and replaces it with a positive statement like 'I will work hard and concentrate on each of my exercises to make it stronger'.

Phase 3: advanced rehabilitation

Cognitive restructuring to address setbacks and goals for a return to sport will be helpful for the injured athlete during the later stages of rehabilitation, and should be incorporated by the therapist as necessary. (For further information about cognitive strategies refer to Chapter 7.)

Social support

Social support refers to an exchange of resources between at least two individuals (e.g. the injured athlete and therapist) to enhance the well-being of the recipient.[44] Research contends that specific types of social support facilitate coping with a particular type of stressful event,[45-47] which emphasizes the need for a matching process between three broad types of social support—emotional, informational, and tangible—and the types of stress encountered during different phases of rehabilitation.

Phase 1: immediate postinjury

The therapist is well positioned to provide the injured athlete with various types of informational, emotional, and tangible support. Informational support from the therapist at this stage is most critical, as it will help to clarify athlete concerns and potentially highlight other issues that may require emotional and tangible support. Social support needs for individual athletes are likely to become apparent to the therapist as treatment continues and the therapist–athlete relationship develops. The therapist should be aware of the important role they play in social support and of some inherent limitations. If the therapist feels uncomfortable with the demands made on them for emotional support from the athlete, it is advisable to investigate possible referral to a sport or clinical psychologist for counseling. For example, therapists may feel they do not have adequate time or the knowledge to help injured athletes, or fear that a dependence relationship could later develop resulting in a negative situation. To assist injured athletes, therapists should encourage the sharing of rehabilitation goals with the support network (e.g. parent/guardian, boyfriend/girlfriend, partner, coach, and other significant others in the athlete's life) so that effective collaboration can take place. The sharing of goals with others should only occur in consultation with the athlete so that his or her informed consent is obtained. Seeking permission to share these goals engenders trust in the therapist and reinforces an internal locus of control within the athlete.

Phase 2: early to progressive rehabilitation

As an active rehabilitation program develops, the therapist can serve an important function by establishing injury support groups, or through peer modelling.[28,48] For example, a support group may operate where other athletes with similar injury problems come together to discuss issues that concern them, or where they meet informally in the clinic as part of their rehabilitation, e.g. for exercise programs. This may be as simple as arranging common appointment times for athletes with similar injuries. Peer modelling involves bringing the injured athlete into contact with another athlete who has recovered successfully from a similar injury.[34] The therapist will be critical to the success of these support plans through networking and co-ordinating the process.

Phase 3: advanced rehabilitation

If the support group and peer modelling strategies are successful, these should continue. Due to the one-on-one nature of the athlete–therapist relationship, the therapist is in an ideal position to assess further support needs and to provide the appropriate assistance. For injuries where a long-term rehabilitation program is required (e.g. significant fractures, or reconstructive surgery of the knee or shoulder), support groups can be an integral part of successful rehabilitation. (For further information about social support refer to Chapter 8.)

Imagery

Imagery has been proposed to assist with pain control, reduce anxiety, and to help develop positive attitudes and self-awareness.[34,37,39,43,49] Imagery is reported to be useful in facilitating the healing process and in promoting a positive outlook toward recovery.[50,51]

Phase 1: immediate postinjury

The technique most useful at this stage of rehabilitation is body rehearsal, which involves the use of healing images, related to successful physical outcomes. The athlete is given a clear description of what has happened internally as a result of the injury and the subsequent process of healing. This information allows the athlete to be able to visualize the healing process taking place, both during treatment and at other times throughout the day. The therapist may help the athlete to create the visual images that can be utilized in the imagery process.[52]

Phase 2: early to progressive rehabilitation

This stage involves progressing the healing images coincident with the appropriate stage of physical recovery. For example, the athlete may visualize the healing of their partially torn knee ligament as 'the knitting together of a finely woven rope where the fibres are interlocked and running in parallel'. The athlete may also find it useful to commence 'coping rehearsal' at this stage, which involves visualizing potential problems or obstacles to recovery and overcoming these successfully. This is regarded as a realistic way of preparing an athlete to deal effectively with setbacks.[53] Coping rehearsal during this phase helps injured athletes to feel more positive about themselves and what they can achieve. Various scenarios can be rehearsed that produce positive feelings such as enthusiasm, pride, and self-confidence.[42,53]

Phase 3: advanced rehabilitation

Mastery rehearsal will be most helpful at this stage, and involves visualizing and rehearsing a successful return to sport. This may also include visualizing the injured area as fully healed, and athletes seeing themselves competing again with no pain or restriction while moving confidently with control. Doing so is likely to promote confidence in the success of rehabilitation and demonstrate a readiness to return to competition. These visual images should also match, and be reinforced by the completion of physical routines that demonstrate the athlete's ability to move confidently with control. (For further information about imagery refer to Chapter 7.)

Confidence training

It is normal for an athlete to experience fears and concerns following injury.[54,55] The provision of information at an appropriate level of understanding, without overloading the athlete, is an important part of rebuilding confidence.

Phase 1: immediate postinjury

The initiation of a goal-setting program will provide a framework for action so the athlete can regain some control, which also has the potential to boost confidence within the athlete and in the athlete–therapist relationship.

Phase 2: early to progressive rehabilitation

Since confidence is affected by the beliefs and thoughts in the mind of injured athletes, the therapist should be vigilant in responding to unrealistic, pessimistic, and irrational beliefs that the athlete may express. Asking specific questions of the injured athlete to elicit how they think and feel in specific situations will often uncover confidence-sapping ideation.[55]

Phase 3: advanced rehabilitation

At this stage, athletes may experience a lack of confidence to return to sport at an acceptable level. There may be a fear of reinjury, or concern about their form or status within the team. Therapists can assist by encouraging athletes to develop positive self-talk and to image success in rehabilitation, management of setbacks, and, ultimately, a successful return to sport.

Implementation and documentation

To be most effective, implementation of periodized psychoeducational strategies should occur within a framework of evidence-based medicine/practice (EBP). The use of EBP focuses on the use of research-based 'best evidence' for the inclusion or prescription of the management of pathology.[56,57] 'Best evidence' is generally founded upon the recency and rigor of published research findings; however, from a patient's perspective 'best practice' may include strategies for care that can be justified with reference to professional judgment in relation to the individual circumstances.[58] Importantly, the use of EBP is also a fundamental way for therapists to satisfy their responsibility in providing the evidence that 'what we do, works'. By planning interventions on 'best evidence' and documenting the process and outcomes, we are in effect contributing to the body of knowledge that allows us to validate what in the past may have been put down as experience as well as providing 'best practice'.

Inherent to providing 'best practice' is the planning of the management of an injury, such that appropriate physical interventions should be assessed immediately as to the outcome, or, within an appropriate time-frame, after the application of the technique or intervention (i.e. increased range of motion, decreased pain, improved gait patterns). This concept can also be applied to interactions within the personal and affective domains. It is not difficult to plan communication and interaction, as well as to ascertain and document the outcome(s) of assistance, in helping the injured athlete to manage the psychological reaction and stresses that may accompany the injury.

The concepts of EBP are easily applied to the use of mental skills training during rehabilitation. Realization, acceptance, and implementation of these concepts will facilitate a more directed and positive outcome for the therapist and the injured athlete by integrating mental skills training within the physical treatment sessions. The essential concepts and processes that can be built into an EBP scheme of management of injured sports persons include:

(1) a clinically reasoned, decision-making process;[59]

(2) knowledge of:

    (a) the choices available for intervention,

    (b) the evidence supporting the intervention,

    (c) the expected outcome of the intervention;

(3) an assessment of the outcome of the intervention;

(4) documentation of:

  (a) the prior state,

  (b) the intervention,

  (c) the outcome;

(5) planning the next progression, based on the outcome of the intervention.

While these concepts and processes are fundamental to the practice of the physical aspects of management, they are also completely relevant to interactions in the affective domain. This approach also fits very neatly with the well-accepted and documented Problem Oriented Medical Record (POMR) approach to record keeping.[60] The ability to record information about the injured athlete's reaction to their injury, as well as documenting environmental factors that may influence the rehabilitation process and the outcome, helps to build the database that is integral to the organization of data centred around the patient's specific complaints.[61] This documentation can follow the 'subjective–objective-assessment plan' (SOAP) approach to recording clinical assessment and management notes.[62,63] It can also be extended to include a more directed 'intervention–evaluation review' (IER)[64] process in recording the results of planned interventions, the outcome of these, and the expected review period during which change might be generally expected to occur. This expanded format then becomes a SOAPIER record, and is used within the three case studies described below. The case studies are typical of situations that a physiotherapist or sports therapist will have already encountered when dealing with injured athletes, across all levels of participation and ages.

In recording the observations both before and after a planned intervention, it is important to only record expressions of behavior and actual dialogue that the client has made, rather than label the athlete or make a diagnosis that therapists are not professionally qualified to make.[63] Therefore, therapists should avoid statements like 'Jane is depressed and has high anxiety levels' or 'John has bouts of paranoia, which when coupled with his introverted personality, makes communication difficult'. These statements may well have been based on several observations and the injured athlete's behavior and expressions, but it is only behaviors and statements that should be recorded. For example, 'Jane told me today that she is not sleeping well and is irritable, and says that she worries a lot about her future sports participation.' Or, 'John says that he is worried that the coach will never play him again in the first team as this is the second time he has been injured before major games. He says that he has few friends in the team and feels that they do not want him in the team.'

Case studies

Case study 1: Phase 1—communication-counseling regarding the grief response

Background: John (age 20) is a club-level soccer player. He has considerable potential and aspires to representative honors. During a preseason game, he suffered a mild knee injury that was diagnosed as a sprain to his left anterior cruciate ligament (ACL). He underwent 5 weeks of physiotherapy treatment for this injury and recently made a successful return to competition. However, yesterday he reinjured his left knee. He was immediately examined by the team doctor and informed that he had ruptured his ACL and would require reconstruction surgery. He was referred to an orthopedic specialist. The result is that this season of competition is over for John. John has been referred to you as a physiotherapist for immediate injury management following the ACL rupture. He appears to be denying the seriousness of his injury.

SOAPIER approach

Subjective: John has made comments like: 'I don't care what the doctor says. I don't have time for surgery and I'm not about to throw away all the hard work I've done so far. I'll be back playing this season.'

Objective: John was observed to immediately isolate himself from his teammates and the coach following this reinjury. He was not seen to discuss the doctor's diagnosis with anyone before packing his gear-bag and leaving the changing rooms. He drove himself to the physiotherapy clinic today and hobbled into the rooms. He appeared somewhat agitated, and expressed his reluctance to accept the doctor's diagnosis.

Assessment: John appears to be denying the seriousness of his injury.

Plan: A full clinical assessment of John's injury needs to be undertaken and John fully briefed as to the findings. Give information in simple language that John can understand and allocate sufficient time to answer all his questions. It may be important to ensure that members of John's support network (e.g. his girlfriend and parents) are present at the next session, to ensure everyone is clear about the seriousness of the injury and the proposed rehabilitation pathway. It is important to make sure there is adequate time for this to occur, and to use aids such as an anatomical knee model and diagrams to help convey information about this injury.

Intervention: Complete a clinical assessment to document the status of the knee and to confirm the doctor's diagnosis of an ACL rupture. Discuss the findings with John, and reinforce with John that he needs to keep his appointment with the orthopedic specialist to obtain direction regarding surgical and non-surgical options. John's questions are to be answered and discussed at a meeting involving his family network at the next visit, which will be scheduled after the specialist consultation expected to take place within the next few days. He expressed keenness to do this and has taken the responsibility to organize for his girlfriend and parents to be present at the next visit.

Evaluation: While not openly willing to accept the seriousness of his injury, John appeared to listen to what was said about the nature of his injury and the consequences of an ACL rupture. He was keen to involve his support network at the next session, which may be important to assist John to cope with this injury. They may be able to help John accept the reality that he is unlikely to compete again this season.

Review: At the next session allow adequate time to discuss the diagnosis again, to follow up on the visit to the specialist, and to answer any questions from John, or his support network. Use models and diagrams again and make explanations as simple as possible. Be aware of anxiety that may be expressed and listen to comments from John that reinforce negative thinking, or his continued lack of acceptance. Such comments will need to be addressed as they arise.

Case study 2: Phase 2—cognitive restructuring

Background: It is mid-season, Dale (age 22) is a representative field hockey player who has a busy schedule ahead of her. For the last two seasons she has had bilateral shin pain that she has found to be very restrictive. To help her manage over this time, she has had regular physiotherapy treatment, but the problem is worsening. Last week she saw an orthopedic specialist for a fresh series of tests and was told that her compartment syndrome had worsened and required surgery. The orthopedic specialist will review her next week and at that time expects to set a date for her surgery. You have always found Dale easy to talk to. She is usually very positive and focused. Hockey means a great deal to her and has her sights set on making the national team. When talking to Dale about the events of the past week you note that she is voicing many concerns.

SOAPIER approach

Subjective: Some of her comments have included:

- 'He [the specialist] doesn't understand what hockey means to me.' 'I can't take time out now. It's just not possible. My career will be ruined.'
- 'I can't believe this is happening to me.'
- 'After he [the specialist] said I needed surgery I went blank. I don't even know what is involved, or how long I'd be out, but what does it matter? No one is going to tell me what to do. It's my body, I'm going to call the shots.'
- 'I don't know about surgery anyway. There is no guarantee he can fix it. Jan (teammate) was telling me a friend of hers had the same surgery and got worse. Given my luck it wouldn't surprise me if the same thing happened to me.'
- 'I'll just 'guts it' out. I'll be right. I can put up with the pain, as long as it's not doing me any long-term damage.'
- 'I'm so pissed off. No one else in the team trains as hard as I do. None of them are as committed as I am and look where I end up. It's not fair.'

Objective: Observed behavior includes that Dale is less positive in her discussions during treatment sessions. She has expressed some degree of hopelessness with her current situation and has even said a number of times: 'Nothing will help!'

However, she does show up on time for her appointments and she reports to be following instructions given for symptomatic management.

Assessment: Conflicting behavior is evident. She is sending a verbal message that says: 'Why bother?' 'What's the point?' A considerable number of negative thoughts are being expressed. Despite this she is compliant with treatment and still appears motivated to continue.

Plan: Need to discuss with Dale the link between her thinking, feelings, and actions. Attempt to restructure her thinking through an awareness of thought-stopping and positive self-talk. Challenge her irrational and catastrophizing thoughts.

Intervention: Spent today's entire session on discussing the specific irrational and catastrophizing thoughts that Dale has repeatedly mentioned. Discussed the thought-stopping technique as a strategy to help identify and change such thinking.

Evaluation: Dale was very receptive to today's discussion about thought-stoppage. She openly acknowledged that lately her thinking has affected her sense of well-being, i.e. she feels she has had less energy because she's been stressed and feeling obligated to make decisions (e.g. surgery) when she's not sure what is involved and what is the likelihood of a favorable outcome. She has confessed that she doesn't want to get her hopes up, so she's been thinking and saying negative things. However, this has not helped and she doesn't believe it is likely to; therefore, she would like to just get on with things and do as much as she can from day-to-day.

Review: Next session, check on Dale's success with recognizing her negative thinking and the use of the thought-stopping technique. If she has grasped this approach then introduce positive self-talk.

Case study 3: Phase 3—lack of confidence to return-to-sport

Background: Anne (age 24) is a competitive basketball player who is rehabilitating from a right ankle injury, which this time has kept her out of competition for 4 weeks. This is the third time this season that she has been sidelined due to this particular ankle problem, and she has expressed some doubts about her ability to return to her preinjury level of fitness and competitive form. Radiological examinations have shown no bony damage or mechanical instability on stress radiographs.

SOAPIER approach

Subjective: Anne has commented: 'My ankle is weak. It will never be the same. Maybe I should just retire now, what is the point of continuing?'

Objective: Anne still has an observable limp at 4 weeks' postinjury. When asked if the ankle is still causing her pain, she insists it is not. However, she appears to noticeably favor it when walking, running, or jumping, particularly when training with others. Otherwise, she does not limp as noticeably when training by herself.

Assessment: Anne has developed a habitual limp and subconsciously is favoring her recurring injured ankle. There are no known physical reasons why she cannot make a full, successful return to sport. But, given her verbal and non-verbal behavior, she appears to be lacking confidence in her physical ability to do so.

Plan: Ensure quality of movement in physical training. Discuss with Anne the physical healing process and the fact there is nothing severe, or a long-term process, that will limit her ability to return to sport at her preinjury level if that is what she would like to do. Answer any questions she has to ensure she is fully informed of the current prognosis and your confidence in her ability to make a full recovery.

Intervention: Set up sport-specific drills for Anne to practice in the rehabilitation clinic. Use a video camera to provide Anne with visual feedback so she can see herself moving. Use models and diagrams to explain the ligamentous damage and repair process to Anne. Answer her questions.

Evaluation: Anne was able to perform the drills without any noticeable limp. She reported that observation of her video was extremely beneficial to assist her with relearning appropriate movement patterns.

Review: Progress sport-specific drills to more complex patterns at faster speeds. Aim to increase physical demands to levels that she will encounter on the basketball court during competition. Discuss the established goal-setting program with Anne. Re-evaluate goals with her so that she is empowered to take control over her return to sport. This may be an important step in the process of rebuilding her confidence.

Summary

The physiotherapist and sport therapist play an integral role in the multidisciplinary sports medicine team. Often, due to the regular contact and the time spent with an injured athlete, they are the health professionals best placed to facilitate positive affective outcomes during the rehabilitation process as well as to identify barriers to success that may require further referral. This chapter has provided:

(1) a framework for the implementation of a periodized 'mental skills training' plan within the rehabilitation process;

(2) the research evidence for the psychoeducational strategies presented; and

(3) demonstrated how these can be integrated within the concepts of evidence-based practice, and how the process can be documented within the SOAPIER approach to problem-oriented, medical record keeping.

References

1. Gordon, S. (1986). Sport psychology and the injured athlete: A cognitive-behavioral approach to injury response and injury rehabilitation. In *Science*

periodical on research and technology in sport. (ed. T. Shevciw) Coaching Association of Canada, Ottawa, Canada.

2. Lavallee, D., Grove, J. R., Gordon, S., and Ford, I. W. (1998). The experience of loss in sport. In *Perspectives on loss: a sourcebook* (ed. J. H. Harvey), pp. 241–52. Bruner/Mazell, Philadelphia, PA.

3. Petitpas, A. Danish, S. J. (1995). Caring for injured athletes. In *Sport psychology interventions* (ed. S. Murphy), pp. 255–81. Human Kinetics, Lower Mitchum, SA.

4. McDonald, S. A. and Hardy, C. J. (1990). Affective response patterns of the injured athlete: An exploratory analysis. *The Sport Psychologist*, **4**, 261–74.

5. Gordon, S., Milios, D., and Grove, J. R. (1991). Psychological aspects of the recovery process from sport injury: The perspective of sport physiotherapists. *Australian Journal of Science and Medicine in Sport*, **23**, 53–60.

6. Taylor, J. and Taylor, S. (1997). *Psychological approaches to sports injury rehabilitation.* Aspen, Gaithersburg, MD.

7. Wiese-Bjornstal, D. M. and Shaffer, S. M. (1999). Psychosocial dimensions of sport injury. In *Counseling in sports medicine* (ed. R. Ray and D. Wiese-Bjornstal), pp. 23–40. Human Kinetics, Champaign, IL.

8. Ford, I. W. and Gordon, S. (1994). Perspectives on the psychological curricula in professional training programs of sport physiotherapists and sport/athletic trainers: a cross-cultural survey. Paper presented at the *Annual meeting of the Association for the Advancement of Applied Sport Psychology*, Lake Tahoe, NV, October 1994.

9. Brewer, B. W., Petitpas, A. J., Van Raalte, J. L., Sklar, J. H., and Ditmar, T. D. (1995). Prevalence of psychological distress among patients at a physical therapy clinic specialising in sports medicine. *Sports Medicine, Training and Rehabilitation*, **6**, 139–45.

10. Larson, G. A., Starkey, C., and Zaichkowsky, L. D. (1996). Psychological aspects of athletic injuries as perceived by athletic trainers. *The Sport Psychologist*, **10**, 37–47.

11. Brewer, B. W., Van Raalte, J. L., and Lindner, D. E. (1991). Role of the sport psychologist in treating injured athletes: A survey of sports medicine providers. *Journal of Applied Sport Psychology*, **3**, 183–90.

12. Gordon, S. and Lindgren, S. (1990). Psycho-physical rehabilitation from a serious sport injury: Case study of an elite fast bowler. *Australian Journal of Science and Medicine in Sport*, **22**, 71–6.

13. Grove, J. R., Stewart, R., and Gordon, S. (1990). Emotional reactions of athletes to knee rehabilitation. Paper presented at the *Annual Scientific Conference of the Australian Sports Medicine Federation*, Alice Springs, Northern Territory, Australia, October 1990.

14. Rose, J. and Jevne, R. F. J. (1993). Psychological processes associated with athletic injuries. *The Sport Psychologist*, **7**, 309–28.

15. Shelley, G. A. (1994). *Athletic injuries: The psychological perspectives of high*

school athletes. Paper presented at the *Annual meeting of the Association for the Advancement of Applied Sport Psychology*, Lake Tahoe, NV, October 1994.

16. Weiss, M. R. and Troxel, R. K. (1986). Psychology of the injured athlete. *Journal of Athletic Training*, **15**, 144–6.

17. Fisher, A. C., Mullins, S. A., and Frye, P. A. (1993). Athletic trainers' attitudes and judgements of injured athletes' rehabilitation adherence. *Journal of Athletic Training*, **28**, 43–7.

18. Wiese, D. M., Weiss, M. R., and Yukelson, D. (1991). Sport psychology in the training room: A survey of athletic trainers. *The Sport Psychologist*, **5**, 15–24.

19. Brewer, B. W., Jeffers, K. E., Petitpas, A. J., and Van Raalte, J. L. (1994). Perceptions of psychological interventions in the context of sport injury rehabilitation. *The Sport Psychologist*, **8**, 176–88.

20. Carroll, S. (1994). Mental imagery as an aid to healing the injured athlete. Paper presented at the *Annual meeting of the Association for the Advancement of Applied Sport Psychology*, Lake Tahoe, NV, October 1994.

21. Ievleva, L. and Orlick, T. (1991). Mental links to enhanced healing: An exploratory study. *The Sport Psychologist*, **5**, 25–40.

22. Lamott, E. E., Petlichkoff, L. M., Van Wassenhove, J., Stein, K., Wade, G., and Lewis, K. (1989). Psychological rehabilitation of the injured athlete: An educational approach to injury. Paper presented at the *Annual meeting of the Association for the Advancement of Applied Sport Psychology*, Seattle, WA, September 1989.

23. Lamott, E. E. and Petlichkoff, L. M. (1990). Psychological factors and the injured athlete: Is there a relationship? Paper presented at the *Annual meeting of the Association for the Advancement of Applied Sport Psychology*, San Antonio, TX, September 1990.

24. Granito, J. V. J., Hogan, J. B., and Varnum, L. K. (1995). The performance enhancement group program: Integrating sport psychology and rehabilitation. *Journal of Athletic Training*, **30**, 328–31.

25. Green, L. B. (1992). The use of imagery in the rehabilitation of injured athletes. *The Sport Psychologist*, **6**, 416–28.

26. Potter, M. and Grove, J. R. (1999). Mental skills training during rehabilitation: Case studies of injured athletes. *New Zealand Journal of Physiotherapy*, **28**, 24–31.

27. Richardson, P. A. and Latuda, L. M. (1995). Therapeutic imagery and athletic injuries. *Journal of Athletic Training*, **30**, 10–12.

28. Striegel, D., Hedgpeth, E., and Sowa, C. (1996). Differential psychological treatment of injured athletes based on length of rehabilitation. *Journal of Sport Rehabilitation*, **5**, 330–5.

29. Wiese-Bjornstal, D. M. and Smith, A. M. (1999). Counseling strategies for enhanced recovery of injured athletes within a team approach. In *Psychological bases of sport injuries* (2nd edn) (ed. D. Pargman), pp. 125–55. Fitness Information Technology, Morgantown, WV.

30. Bassett, S. F. and Petrie, K. J. (1999). The effect of treatment goals on patient compliance with physiotherapy exercise programs. *Physiotherapy*, **85**, 130–7.
31. DePalma, M. T. and DePalma, B. (1989). The use of instruction and the behavioral approach to facilitate injury rehabilitation. *Journal of Athletic Training*, **24**, 217–19.
32. Wiese-Bjornstal, D. M., Gardetto, D. M., and Shaffer, S. M. (1999). Effective interaction skills for sports medicine professionals. In *Counseling in sports medicine* (ed. R. Ray and D. Wiese-Bjornstal), pp. 55–74. Human Kinetics, Champaign, IL.
33. Cott, C. and Finch, E. (1990). Goal-setting in physical therapy practice. *Physiotherapy Canada*, **43**, 19–22.
34. Wiese, D. M. and Weiss, M. R. (1987). Psychological rehabilitation and physical injury: Implications for the sports medicine team. *The Sport Psychologist*, **1**, 318–30.
35. Gilbourne, D. (1996). Goal-setting during injury rehabilitation. In *Science and soccer* (ed. T. Reilly), pp. 185–200. E. and F. N. Spon, London.
36. Ermler, K. L. and Thomas, C. E. (1990). Interventions for the alienating effect of injury. *Journal of Athletic Training*, **25**, 269–71.
37. Porter, K. and Foster, J. (1987). Who will stop the pain? Overcome your injuries with a program of positive imagery. *World Tennis*, **35**, 28–30.
38. Pearson, L. and Jones, G. (1992). Emotional effects of sports injuries: Implications for physiotherapists. *Physiotherapy*, **78**, 762 70.
39. Singer, R. N. and Johnson, P. J. (1987). Strategies to cope with pain associated with sport-related injuries. *Journal of Athletic Training*, **22**, 100–3.
40. Lichstein, K. L. (1988). *Clinical relaxation strategies*. Wiley, New York.
41. Hardy, L. (1992). Psychological stress, performance and injury in sport. *British Medical Bulletin*, **48**, 615–29.
42. Yukelson, D. (1986). Psychology of sports and the injured athlete. In *Sports physical therapy* (ed. D. B. Bernhardt), pp. 173–95. Churchill Livingston, New York.
43. Grove, J. R. and Gordon, A. M. D. (1995). The psychological aspects of injury in sport. In *Textbook of science and medicine in sport* (2nd edn) (ed. J. Bloomfield, P. A. Fricker, and K. D. Fitch), pp. 194–205. Blackwell, Melbourne, Australia.
44. Shumaker, S. A. and Brownell, A. (1984). Toward a theory of social support: Closing conceptual gaps. *Journal of Social Issues*, **40**, 11–36.
45. Hardy, C. J. and Crace, R. K. (1993). The dimensions of social support when dealing with sport injuries. In *Psychological bases of sports injuries* (ed. D. Pargman), pp. 121–44. Fitness Information Technology, Morgantown, WV.
46. Thoits, P. A. (1995). Stress, coping, and social support processes: Where are we? What next? *Journal of Health and Social Behavior* (extra issue), 53–79.
47. Udry, E. (1997). Coping and social support among injured athletes following surgery. *Journal of Sport and Exercise Psychology*, **19**, 71–90.

48. Pargman, D. (1999). *Psychological bases of sport injury* (2nd edn). Fitness Information Technology, Morgantown, WV.

49. Feltz, D. (1986). The psychology of sports injuries. In *Sports injuries: the unthwarted epidemic* (ed. P. F. Vinger and E.G. Hoerner), pp. 336–44). P. S. G. Publishing Company, Littleton, MA.

50. Green, L. B. (1999). The use of imagery in the rehabilitation of injured athletes. In *Psychological bases of sport injuries* (ed. D. Pargman), pp. 235–51. Fitness Information Technology, Morgantown, WV.

51. Warner, L. and McNeill, M. E. (1988). Mental imagery and its potential for physical therapy. *Physical Therapy,* **68**, 516–21.

52. Heil, J. (1993). *Psychology of sport injury*. Human Kinetics, Champaign, IL.

53. Williams, J. M., Rotella, R. J., and Heyman, S. R. (1998). Stress, injury, and the psychological rehabilitation of athletes. In *Applied sport psychology: personal growth to peak performance* (2nd edn) (ed. J. M. Williams), pp. 409–28. Mayfield, London.

54. Ford, I. W. and Gordon, S. (1998). Guidelines for using sport psychology in rehabilitation. *Athletic Therapy Today*, 3, 41–4.

55. Horsley, C. (1995). Understanding and managing the injured athlete. In *Sports physiotherapy: applied science and practice* (ed. M. Zuluaga, C. Briggs, J. Carlisle, *et al.*), pp. 297–314. Churchill Livingstone, Melbourne, Australia.

56. Sackett, D. L., Rosenberg, W. M., Gray, J. A., Haynes, R. B., and Richardson, W. S. (1996). Evidence based medicine: What it is and what it isn't. *British Medical Journal,* **312**, 71–2. [Editorial]

57. Straus, S. E. and Sackett, D. L. (1998). Using research findings in clinical practice. *British Medical Journal,* **317**, 339–42.

58. Greenhalgh, T. (1999). Narrative based medicine: Narrative based medicine in an evidence based world. *British Medical Journal,* **318**, 323–5.

59. Higgs, J. and Jones, M. (1995). *Clinical reasoning in the health professions*. Butterworth–Heinemann, Boston, MA.

60. Weed, L. L. (1969). *Medical records, medical education, and patient care: The problem-oriented record as a basic tool*. Case Western Reserve University Press, Cleveland, OH.

61. Berni, R. and Readey, H. (1978). *Problem-oriented medical record implementation: allied health peer review* (2nd edn). Mosby, St Louis, MO.

62. Kettenbach, G. (1995). *Writing SOAP notes* (2nd edn). F. A. Davis, Philadelphia, PA.

63. Ray, R. (1999). Documentation in counseling. In *Counseling in sports medicine* (ed. R. Ray and D. Wiese-Bjornstal), pp. 143–60. Human Kinetics, Champaign, IL.

64. Anonymous (1999). Using SOAP, SOAPIE, and SOAPIER formats. *Nursing,* **29**, 75.

5 *Coping strategies*

Gretchen A. Kerr and Patricia S. Miller

Introduction

We know intuitively that there are tremendous individual differences in the way people appraise and cope with life stressors. One only needs to consider Holocaust survivors to appreciate the human potential to overcome extraordinary levels of stress. And yet, others suffer deleterious consequences with relatively minor stressors. Physicians speak freely of the influence of patients' attitudes, particularly optimism and pessimism, on the course of illness. Some patients, after receiving a diagnosis of terminal illness, defy the odds and do not succumb, while others die relatively quickly, particularly if they welcome death for religious reasons.[1] Similarly, with reference to sport, athletes vary substantially in the ways in which they cope with injury;[2-4] some recover more quickly than the physician predicted, while others malinger. In the more extreme case of career-ending injuries, some athletes respond with depression and despair and others navigate the transition to new careers with confidence. These individual differences in responses to stress have provided impetus for the study of coping strategies.

This chapter will address the functions and types of coping strategies with reference to athletic injury. Furthermore, the mediating factors that affect the choice and efficacy of various coping strategies will be discussed. Finally, recommendations will be made for future research and for enhancing the coping process for injured athletes.

Definitions of coping

Coping may be defined as the cognitive and behavioural efforts used by an individual to decrease the effects of stress.[5] Lazarus and Folkman (see ref. 6, p.141 therein) elaborate with the following definition: '...constantly changing cognitive and behavioral efforts to manage specific external and/or internal demands that are appraised as taxing or exceeding the resources of the person'. There are three important features of this definition. First, coping is referred to as a process in which the thoughts and behaviours of an individual are considered within a specific context at a specific point in time. In this way, one's thoughts and behaviours may change continuously as the stressful encounter unfolds. In the case of athletic injury, the athlete's thoughts and behaviours will differ from the time of injury occurrence, throughout the recovery process, to the point of re-entry to sport participation. Second, the coping process is contextual; it must be viewed in terms of the specific context encountered. This transactional perspective,[1,6] which assumes that the individual, situation, and the coping mechanism mutually affect each other in a process that evolves over time, is reflected in the contemporary literature on coping. In this way, an injured athlete's coping will depend upon the interactions of such factors as the severity of injury, personality of the athlete, and support systems available. And third, the potential confounds between the coping process and the outcome or success of coping are averted by referring only to the efforts needed to manage the situation. The hallmark of coping strategies is that they require effort, whether conscious or unconscious, to manage stressful situations and emotional distress.[1] Consequently, coping includes anything a person thinks or does regardless of how well or badly it works.[6]

Functions of coping

Numerous researchers have proposed that there are different functions or objectives of coping. One researcher[7] for example, described the multiple functions of coping as follows:

(1) to secure information about the environment;

(2) to maintain satisfactory internal conditions for both action and for processing information; and

(3) to maintain autonomy or freedom to use one's repertoire in a flexible fashion.

According to others,[8] the functions of coping are to: modify the circumstances giving rise to stress; manage the meaning of circumstances, cognitively and perceptually, to minimize their potency; and to control and relieve the symptoms of distress. In each of these examples, coping serves both to manage external demands or stressors and to maintain a certain level of internal, psychological equilibrium.

Types of coping strategies

To achieve the functions or objectives of coping, researchers have proposed a number of coping strategies or techniques. Researchers have, for example, identified six types of coping strategies,[9] including:

(1) avoidance (doing things to take your mind off the situation);

(2) positive reappraisal (thinking about a situation in a different way to reduce distress);

(3) religion (relying on religious beliefs);

(4) active coping (thinking of possible ways to improve the situation);

(5) active behavioural (doing things to improve the situation); and

(6) social support (talking to others about the situation).

Similarly, Stone and Neale[10] proposed coping strategies of direct action, seeking social support, reinterpretation of the situation, distraction, acceptance, tension release, catharsis, and prayer. While the terminology used in these various frameworks differs slightly, there are clear similarities. In all models of stress and coping, whether stated explicitly or implicitly, there are two types or categories of coping strategies. These have been coined by Lazarus and Folkman[6] as problem-focused coping and emotion-focused coping. This distinction between problem-focused and emotion-focused coping is the most widely accepted conceptualization of coping strategies. Each of these will be addressed in turn.

One function or objective of coping is to manage, regulate, or alter the problem that is causing distress. This is termed problem-focused coping[6] and includes strategies that are directed both at the environment and inwardly on the self. Examples of strategies focused primarily on the environment include altering environmental barriers and resources, such as joining a weight-control programme. Problem-focused strategies that are directed at the self include reducing ego involvement, shifting one's level of aspiration, finding alternative channels of gratification, and learning new skills such as time management and goal-setting.[11]

Folkman and Lazarus[12] developed 'The Ways of Coping Checklist' to assess problem-focused and emotion-focused coping. On the basis of statistical clustering analyses of the items on the checklist, three subcategories of problem-focused coping strategies were identified. These included: confrontational coping (aggressive efforts to change the situation); planful problem-solving (deliberate problem-focused efforts to solve the situation); support seeking (enlisting the help of others to problem-solve). Samples of these items are found in Table 5.1.

A second function of coping is to maintain a level of psychological equilibrium. This is termed emotion-focused coping and refers to cognitive and behavioural efforts to regulate emotional responses to distress. Cognitive efforts such as social comparisons, avoidance, minimization, 'looking at the bright side', cognitive reframing, and selective attention, are often used to reduce distress through changing the meaning of a situation. Behaviours such as engaging in exercise, meditating, alcohol and drug consumption, religion, venting anger, and seeking social support[6] are often pursued to make one feel better. Emotion-focused coping is thought to reduce distress through

Table 1   Sample items from the Ways of Coping Checklist[12]

Problem-focused coping strategies	Emotion-focused coping strategies
Confrontational coping 'I stood my ground and fought for what I wanted.'	*Distancing* 'I went on as if nothing had happened.'
Planful problem-solving 'I made a plan of action and followed it.'	*Self-control* 'I tried to keep my feelings to myself.'
Seeking social support (problem-focused) 'I talked to someone who could do something concrete about the problem.'	*Accepting responsibility* 'I realized I brought the problem on myself.'
	Escape-avoidance 'I tried to make myself feel better by eating, drinking, smoking, etc.'
	Positive reappraisal 'I changed or grew as a person in a good way.'
	Seeking social support (emotion-focused) 'I accepted sympathy and emotional support from someone.'

the maintenance of hope and optimism, denial of facts and the implications of these facts, and the protection of the 'psychological economy of the person'.[6]

The Ways of Coping Checklist includes the following subcategories of emotion-focused coping: positive reappraisal (efforts to find a positive meaning in the experience by focusing on personal growth), distancing (efforts to detach oneself from the stressful situation), accepting responsibility (acknowledging one's role in the problem), self-control (efforts to regulate one's feelings), and escape or avoidance (efforts to escape or avoid the situation by eating, drinking, smoking, using drugs or medications). Samples of these items are found in Table 5.1.

It appears that people use both problem-focused and emotion-focused coping strategies in most situations to control stress levels.[13] However, the nature of the stressor determines which strategy is used predominantly. Furthermore, coping strategies have differential effectiveness depending upon the nature of the situation.

Research consistently indicates that problem-focused coping is more likely to be used and to be more efficacious when people appraise themselves as having control, power, or responsibility in a particular situation or role. For example, several researchers[14] found that problem-focused coping predicted a reduction in depression only when the situation was appraised as changeable. Conversely, those who used emotion-focused coping with changeable events become more depressed. Therefore, individuals who addressed their emotions when they could have managed the problem fared poorly. Other researchers similarly reported that uncontrollable stressors were best handled with emotion-focused coping, [15] whereas problem-focused coping was more helpful with controllable stressors. In other words, when an intervention is needed, problem-focused coping is called for. [16] It follows therefore, that an injured athlete who has control over whether she/he returns to full participation, would be best served through problem-focused coping strategies such as seeking medical advice, adhering to the rehabilitation programme, and setting goals for rehabilitation. Adaptive coping also includes knowing when to stop trying to achieve a goal that is unattainable. If full recovery is impossible, it would be important for adaptive reasons for the injured athlete to refocus efforts to adjusting to his or her 'new' physical state.

When a situation is not changeable and acceptance is required, as in the case of a career-ending injury, emotion-focused coping is more efficacious. [16] In such instances, the emotional responses can still be altered to reduce feelings of distress. As an example, an injured athlete may reframe the situation in a positive manner by thinking, 'My athletic career may be over, but I have other interests and skills that are transferable to a new career'. This athlete may also reduce emotional distress by engaging in such emotion-focused behaviours as seeking support from other athletes who have had their careers terminated prematurely, or by talking through his/her anger, disappointment, and frustration.

It should be mentioned that emotion-focused coping and problem-focused coping can be mutually facilitative. For example, an injured athlete may use problem-focused coping to adhere to the rehabilitation programme and emotion-focused coping to manage the emotional distress associated with the recovery process. However, these forms of coping can also impede one another. An athlete who has experienced a mild concussion, ignores medical advice, and resumes play would be an example.

The match between the demands of a situation and the coping strategies used by the individual is termed 'goodness of fit' [17] and affects the efficacy of coping strategies. An athlete who has incurred a career-ending injury may demonstrate 'goodness of fit' by saying: 'I can't change the fact that my athletic career is over, but I can change how I feel about it'. In this way, the use of emotion-focused coping reduces distress and still leaves the athlete in control. A poor fit would exist if an athlete with a career-ending injury continued to build his/her life around an athletic career, thereby exacerbating feelings of frustration and distress. On the other hand, an injured athlete who has the potential to recover fully, and does not engage in problem-focused coping by adhering to rehabilitation, is also an example of a poor fit.

Mediators

Conceptual models of psychological response to sport injury have identified personal and situational factors as mediators in the coping and rehabilitation processes.[18–20] In other words, the efficacy of coping strategies and 'goodness of fit' seem to depend upon a number of personal and situational factors.[21, 22] Personal mediators have included self-esteem, locus of control, and the type of injury. Factors such as social support, level of competition, and access to rehabilitation have been subsumed under situational mediators. However, Kaplan[13] cautions against the separation of situational from personal mediators. Congruent with the transactional perspective described earlier, the person and situation or environment are continuously interacting with and exerting influence on one another. For example, social support, which has traditionally been viewed as an environmental resource, is now, more and more, recognized as an internal resource because the ability to perceive and make use of social support depends in part on personality, social competence, and self-disclosure skills. Similarly, self-esteem, traditionally thought of as an internal, personal factor, is heavily influenced by messages from one's environment.

We have chosen to focus on the following mediating factors that have received significant attention in the sport injury literature: timing of injury occurrence, type and severity of injury, injury history, personality, appraisal, gender, and context. These will be presented in three categories including: characteristics of the injury; characteristics of the athlete; and characteristics of the context. Recognizing that one category of mediators undoubtedly affects another, each will be addressed in turn.

Characteristics of the injury

Type of injury

The type of injury, distinguished along several different continua in the literature, is believed to have a significant effect on athletes' reactions to and recovery from sport injuries.[23–26] Flint[23] categorized injuries based on their onset as either macro- or microtrauma, with the former defined as injuries stemming from a sudden discrete impact and the latter as the accumulation of repetitive, seemingly negligible, damage. Corresponding distinctions include acute versus chronic injuries,[27] acute versus recurring injuries,[26] and acute versus gradual injuries.[28]

Athletes who suffer macrotrauma or acute injuries can target the explicit cause of their injuries, which may help them deal more effectively with psychological reactions, as well as clearly directing their rehabilitation efforts. Alternatively, athletes who have endured discomfort over a prolonged period may be in greater danger of experiencing difficult psychological and emotional reactions when the pain becomes intolerable. Athletes who have sustained acute injuries may be unprepared to cope with the associated pain and consequences, yet able to quickly access coping resources including meaningful social support.[28] Athletes afflicted with microtrauma or chronic injuries, however, often become accustomed to coping with discomfort and are probably quite adept at ignoring or disregarding pain.[28] Likewise, people in an athlete's social support network may have difficulty recognizing and responding to an escalated chronic injury that the athlete has been able to deal with adequately on his/her own for an extended period.

Practitioners[27] investigated the effect of chronic versus acute injuries on athletes' self-esteem and coping behaviours using the Rosenberg Self-Esteem Inventory and several subscales of the Ways of Coping Questionnaire. Chronically injured athletes scored significantly higher on 'Escape/avoidance' and significantly lower on 'Seeking social support' than athletes with acute injuries. No difference emerged on the 'Accepting responsibility' subscale. The findings confirmed that chronically injured athletes exhibit significantly different coping behaviours than athletes with acute injuries.

Injuries have also been differentiated into three distinct categories according to their course over time: progressive, constant, and episodic injuries.[28] Progressive injuries manifest themselves in continuous, predictable steps toward either recovery or permanent disability. Their course is stable and gradual, requiring athletes to make a series of adaptations to changing levels of health and mobility. The length of recovery and adaptation may vary, meaning that the coping period may be prolonged, yet the predictable nature of the course of the injury typically alleviates some psychological and emotional distress. Problem-focused coping strategies are clearly indicated with progressive injuries, particularly with reference to the course of rehabilitation. However, emotion-focused coping strategies may also have a role to play with progressive injuries, especially if the injury is serious and the onset was unanticipated.

Injuries classified as constant, mean that the level of health and mobility will not differ significantly with the passage of time. Athletes must therefore cope with a new level of physical ability that may involve adapting to a new athletic position, finding a sport tailored to their present physical capacities, or discontinuing participation in sport altogether.[28] Constant-course injuries may require exceptional coping abilities over a protracted period, and may therefore be a significant strain on coping resources. A favourable recovery depends on the degree to which the athlete and his/her support network can successfully adjust to the new level of physical ability. As the athlete has less control over these types of injury, emotion-focused coping strategies such as positive reappraisal and seeking emotional support are likely to be more efficacious, although this supposition has yet to be tested.

Episodic or relapsing injuries are characterized by alternating symptom-free and relapse periods. Athletes are in a continuous state of uncertainty regarding recurrence, a condition that taxes coping capacities and interferes with recovery.[28] With these injuries, problem-focused coping may be useful in preventing relapses, while emotion-focused strategies may help with the uncertainty that must be endured. It is hoped that future research will address these possibilities.

Injury severity

Whether an injury causes slight or severe damage will undoubtedly influence coping responses and recovery. Injury severity has been recognized as an important mediating factor in the injury coping process, although delimiting the specific degrees of severity has been difficult.[23] Researchers and practitioners have used diverse means to assess the severity of an injury, with the most common methods being time loss, pain measures, range of motion, and disability. There is considerable variability in the use of these measures, confounding the comparison between studies and the consolidation of findings.

None the less, professionals have made a number of assertions regarding the influence of injury severity on coping and recovery. It is generally accepted that the more severe the injury, the greater the psychological and emotional response and more serious and prolonged the entreaty for coping resources.[4] Athletes who have endured a serious injury requiring withdrawal from sport for a significant period, respond initially with shock and denial and often harbour a false belief that the injury is superficial.[24] Psychological trauma such as emotional distress, identity loss, fear, anxiety, and challenges to self-confidence, have also been added to the list of responses to severe sport injuries.[28] Athletes with severe injuries, defined as being prohibited from sport for more than two weeks, exhibited significant mood disturbance, while those with mild and moderate injuries displayed less mood disturbance than the general, non-injured population.[29] Likewise, injury severity emerged as a significant predictor of postinjury depression[30] among male and female competitive athletes suffering acute injuries.

It should be stressed that most athletes cope well with their sport injuries and that their clinical reactions are limited, as indicated by a relative absence of depression and general emotional distress.[3] A small percentage of athletes do, however, experience emotional, psychological, and behavioural distress necessitating clinical intervention. Practitioners have suggested that young athletes suffering acute injuries and who lacked perceived support for or control over rehabilitation are most vulnerable to postinjury distress.[3] A second group of practitioners[31] similarly noted that those most at risk for suicide attempts postinjury are young, seriously injured athletes, who exhibited clinical depression scores, required surgery, and were unlikely to return to preinjury levels of participation where they had once enjoyed meaningful success. These two studies suggest that the athlete's age may be an important mediator of coping responses. While very few athletes require clinical intervention following a sport injury, healthcare professionals and significant figures in the lives of athletes need to recognize extreme responses to injury and the imposed withdrawal from sport.

Season and career-ending injuries

These injuries warrant special attention in any discussion of coping strategies for injured athletes. Athletes who suffer a season or career-ending injury appear to experience greater difficulty coping with their injury and have a greater tendency to exhibit dysfunctional coping behaviours such as substance abuse. Excessive levels of stress, like those aroused by career-ending injuries, are more likely to create emotional distress and therefore require emotion-focused coping strategies. Indeed, research has supported the positive relationship between the degree of stress experienced and reliance on emotion-focused coping strategies.[32] Furthermore, severe stressors seem to inhibit problem-focused coping through detrimental effects on cognitive functioning and the capacity for information-processing. Ineffective information gathering and evaluation may lead to obsessive thoughts, constricted cognitive functioning, and premature closure on decisions.[6] Physicians, for example, tend to recognize the compromising effects of distress on problem-solving abilities when giving bad news to patients. The patient's ability to absorb all the information is impaired and, thus, the perceptive physician allows time to adjust to a diagnosis before giving information about treatment and procedures.[6] The inability to perceive and process such disturbing information may account for the initial denial often observed in many injured athletes. Denial has been cited as a typical first response to severe stressors, including athletic injury. It appears that initial denial can be an important and effective adaptive response to crises when the situation cannot yet be faced in its entirety. Rutter[33] also reported that immediately after the stressful life event, avoidance strategies could be effective in reducing distress. Over the long-term however, approach strategies were more effective. Therefore, the amount of time that has elapsed since the start of the problem influences the effectiveness of various strategies. Similarly, the healthcare provider can afford to approach minor problems with a 'threat minimization' or 'wait and see' strategy, an approach that would be unlikely to be effective with more major problems[1] such as a career-ending injury.

There have been a number of cases of Olympic, professional, and university athletes with career-ending injuries who reportedly suffered depression and engaged in emotion-focused coping strategies such as alcohol and drug abuse as responses to their injuries.[28] Without control over the premature end to their careers, problem-focused coping strategies are ineffective, thus leaving the athlete to rely exclusively on emotion-focused coping. Practitioners discovered that college student-athletes who had suffered a career-ending injury expressed significantly lower levels of life satisfaction than non-injured peers from 3 to 8 years after graduation.[34] The lower levels of life satisfaction evident after such long periods may have been related to feelings of unfinished business or unfulfilled dreams.

Coping responses and recovery are further exacerbated when the athlete's identity and ego are heavily dependent on the athlete role. Research indicates that the more central the area is to one's value system and identity, the more distress is experienced when threats or harm arise in that area.[35] As such, if an individual defines himself or herself solely, or even primarily, as an athlete, then a career-ending injury will probably create substantial distress. If, on the other hand, the athlete defines himself or herself in many other ways in addition to being an athlete, then a career-ending injury does not have the same impact for one's identity or future career choices. Here is an illustrative example of the interplay between an environmental mediator of a career-ending injury and a personal mediator of identity.

A number of suggestions for helping athletes cope with season-ending injuries based on empirical research and applied work with injured athletes are available. Researchers drew upon in-depth interviews with male and female elite skiers who had suffered injuries that prevented the completion of a competitive season or forced the athlete to withdraw from participation for a minimum of 3 months.[36] Recommendations for assisting injured athletes were divided into distinct categories and included: educate and inform; use appropriate motivation; demonstrate empathy and support; facilitate positive interactions; augment athletes' confidence; and provide customized training. In addition, injured athletes preferred healthcare providers with likeable personalities and a demonstrated level of competence. These recommendations refer to the two functions of coping—enhancing the athletes' recovery, and reducing or managing their feelings of distress.

Timing of the injury

The timing of various coping strategies is also important in dealing with stressors. Research has shown that the timing of an injury across the athletic season may influence athletes' coping responses and subsequent recovery.[23,24] The number of games or events that will be missed during rehabilitation, the proximity of the injury to important events, and the remaining number of games or events in a season will affect the injury-coping process. Athletes forced to withdraw from a significant number of games or events due to sport injuries are more likely to express emotional and psychological distress. Similarly, athletes' reactions may be intensified when prohibited from major competitions, particularly qualifying or championship events, due to sport injuries. Forced to the sidelines for an event that an athlete has prepared for over an extended period or had anticipated would propel his/her athletic career can be extremely discouraging. Again, the importance of emotion-focused coping is highlighted here.

Quinn and Fallon,[37] in their examination of changes in the psychological reactions of injured athletes throughout their rehabilitation, found that athletes used active coping strategies such as planning, initiating direct action, and increasing their efforts. The researchers also found that the use of coping strategies remained relatively stable over time. While the use of active coping strategies such as problem-solving increased slightly over time, there was no change in the use of passive coping strategies, such as denial, over the course of rehabilitation.

Characteristics of the athlete

Personality

Research has shown that personality traits such as self-esteem, locus of control, and neuroticism affect the use of coping strategies and coping effectiveness. For example, individuals with an internal locus of control and a high self-esteem tend to use more problem-focused coping and less emotion-focused coping strategies than those with an external locus of control and low self-esteem. More recently, the literature has suggested that those with an internal locus of control, high self-esteem, and low neuroticism have the flexibility or repertoire to use the coping strategy most suited to the situation.[32]

Taylor and Aspinwall[16] reported that university students with high self-esteem and a sense of optimism used higher levels of active coping strategies and were less likely to avoid their difficulties through daydreaming, drinking, or isolating themselves. Similarly, Stanton and Snider[38] found that optimism predicted lower levels of avoidance-coping among women anticipating a potential diagnosis of breast cancer. In turn, avoidance-coping predicted a greater negative mood both pre- and postbiopsy. A sense of optimism has been found to be related to psychological and physical well-being in many ways,[39] but has yet to be investigated in terms of athletic injury.

One could speculate that if stable coping styles or personality traits exist, then similar coping responses would be observed regardless of the situation. However, research has shown that the extent to which cross-situational consistency in coping exists depends upon whether people are responding to similar types of situations. More specifically, the similarity of the appraisals affects the degree to which responses generalize across situations.[32]

Gender

Research has found that the choice of coping strategies is also influenced by gender. The work of Thoits[40] and Gilligan[41] suggest that women are more likely to use an expressive style of coping, which includes such behaviours as seeking social support, writing about the situation, and expressing feelings. Conversely, men tend to analyse or think through a situation, and accept the situation, a style that Thoits refers to as rational or stoic. It is a consistent finding that women use a greater number of coping strategies.

Appraisal

Coping is largely determined by one's appraisal or the meaning one gives to a particular event. Even with extreme negative stressors such as the death of a loved one, appraisals can vary. This particular event will have different meanings depending on whether it involved the accidental, unexpected death of a young, healthy person or the anticipated death of an elderly, ill person. Cognitive appraisal models have been more effective in accounting for individual differences than have stage models.[42] Similarly, the appraisal of an athletic injury may vary considerably. For some, an injury may not be appraised as being stressful or negative; instead, an injury may be a relief to a small number of athletes. Indirect benefits can stem from the maintenance of the injury and the imposed withdrawal from sport. Athletes who are injured may receive attention from coaches, teammates, family, and friends, in addition to material gains and assistance with daily chores. Injured athletes receive a reprieve from training; athletes who are struggling with their performance, who experience intense sport-related anxiety, or those who are considering leaving sport may see an injury as a reprieve from sport altogether. Practitioners noted that these types of secondary gains should not be overlooked in the response to and recovery from sport injuries.[28]

In the case of career-ending injuries, these may be appraised as a 'fall from heaven' for athletes who are enjoying their sport experience and have unfulfilled goals or a 'rescue from hell'[35] for those who have lost the drive and passion for sport. The coping strategies employed in these two instances cannot be equated simply because the same stressor, a career-ending injury, is experienced in both scenarios. In fact, appraisal has been found to be a better predictor of coping responses than the nature of the situation itself.[32] It is important therefore, for healthcare providers to ascertain the meaning of the injury for the athlete.

Characteristics of the context

Injury history

An athlete's injury history will influence his/her coping response to sport injuries. Athletes who have never suffered an injury may respond quite differently to those who have sustained multiple injuries during their athletic careers. Athletes injured for the first time may be unfamiliar with the pain and discomfort associated with injury and impaired mobility. They may be uncertain about their injury prognosis and the rehabilitation process, including which sensations and reactions are normal and which require supplementary medical attention.[23, 28] In addition, athletes coping with a sport injury for the first time may question their ability to recover from the injury and their likelihood of returning to their preinjury performance levels. Without knowledge of the injury and rehabilitation processes and without prior success in overcoming a sport injury, athletes injured for the first time may experience greater fear and anxiety than multiple-injured peers. Indeed, Johnson[43] found that athletes injured for the first time experienced psychological difficulties following long-term injuries, including less confidence, greater stress during the rehabilitation period, and disrupted mood in comparison with athletes who had suffered multiple injuries. Emotion-focused coping strategies appear to be indicated here.

As the coping responses of athletes injured for the first time may differ significantly from peers with a history of sport injuries, their needs may also vary. The newly injured athlete may benefit from information about the injury, the rehabilitation process, and the probability of full recovery. Education relating to the anatomy of the injury, expected and imposed functional restrictions, and rehabilitation protocols would be helpful,[44] as would reassurances of the effectiveness of physical therapy and the importance of adherence to rehabilitation programmes. These are important implications for the healthcare provider.

At the other end of the spectrum are athletes who have suffered multiple sport injuries. Their response will undoubtedly be affected by previous injury trauma and the effectiveness, or lack thereof, of former rehabilitation strategies.[24] Athletes with a history of physical and psychological trauma stemming from sport injuries, athletes with a history of poor coping, and athletes discouraged by past rehabilitation programmes may be at increased risk of deleterious and protracted responses to subsequent injuries.

Other stressors

Although difficult to account for, understanding the impact of one stressful life event, such as an injury, depends heavily on the backdrop of major and minor stressors against which the injury occurs. Coping is not disconnected from what has gone before or what is anticipated for the future.[45] As Pearlin (see ref. 35, p.263 therein) writes, 'We should not assume, as we often do, that because people share one stressful circumstance that we happen to be observing that they are therefore alike with regard to their total exposure to stressors.' Chronic strain, for example, appears to exacerbate the impact of stressful life events, particularly when they occur within the same or related domains.[16] In this way, if an athlete has been experiencing ongoing frustrations with his/her performance and resultant interpersonal difficulties with the coaches, the impact of an injury will probably be accentuated. Conversely, in some instances, stressful events may have a lessened impact if they pale in comparison to other stressors, particularly when they occur in unrelated domains. So, an injury to an athlete may have less psychological impact if he/she is dealing simultaneously with the death of a parent.

Medical practitioners also need to consider the constellation or cascade of primary and secondary stressors associated with stressful events.[35] A primary stressor such as divorce, for example, may lead to a cascade of secondary stressors such as a move to a less desirable residence, financial strain, and adjustment difficulties with children. For the athlete facing a career-ending injury, secondary stressors could include a loss of income and support network, identity confusion, and uncertainty about another career. On the other hand, positive cascades of secondary events are possible. For the athlete for whom the career-ending injury provides relief, positive secondary events could include moving on to a more permanent career, the next stage of life-span development, and in general, a more balanced lifestyle.

One's appraisal, coping efforts, and resistance and vulnerability to stress are influenced by such factors as time, money, socioeconomic status, social support, and the presence or absence of other life stressors. For example, Booth and Amato[46] found that following divorce, both men and women with higher incomes, educational attainment, and more friends, experienced less distress. With respect to working mothers, having a flexible work environment and a high degree of control tends to ease the strains associated with combining employment and child-rearing.[47] Norris and Murrell[48] reported that the resources of health, self-esteem, social support, education, and urban lifestyle did not affect the likelihood of experiencing stressful events, but did mute the impact of these stressors when they occurred. However, as the amount of stress increased, the coping advantage provided by these resources lessened, suggesting that, at a critical point, stress may overwhelm even the most protective factors. Medical practitioners may enhance their roles by learning about the broader context in which athletes live and train.

Sport ethic

The broader context of sport or 'sport ethic'[49] must be addressed when considering the coping responses of injured athletes. Research indicates that athletes accept the risk of injury as inherent to sport, consequently they may ignore pain and discomfort and avoid seeking medical attention for injuries. Nixon[50-54] has written about a culture of sport that glorifies playing 'through' injuries, normalizes pain and risk, and heavily pressures athletes to return to competition before they are completely recovered. According to Nixon, many athletes play while injured, return to sport well before they are healed, and are exposed to intense pressure from coaches, teammates, and even athletic trainers to compete while hurt.[52,53] Many coaches are ambivalent to the pain and injury experiences of athletes and expect athletes to take risks with their short- and long-term physical health. Few significant figures in the lives of athletes discourage them from playing while injured or prioritize the short- and long-term health of the athletes over more immediate competitive goals.

This culture of pain and injury saturates high-level sport in North America. Researchers found physical risk central to the sport experiences of male athletes who were willing and encouraged to play while injured.[55] Disassociative strategies were used to cope with injuries, including denying, disregarding, and depersonalizing pain and injured body parts. These strategies were similarly utilized by female athletes who were equally willing to expose themselves to risk and injury and who were as likely to be exposed to pressure to play aggressively or while injured.[56] It can be seen here that problem-focused and emotion-focused coping strategies can be used to quite a different end or outcome than recovery from injury.

Medical practitioners, coaches, and others in support roles are encouraged to consider their own views of risk, pain, and injury in sport and the degree to which their attitudes about sport contribute to this culture of risk and pain and thus affect the short- and long-term health of athletes.

Other mediating factors

A list of additional potential mediating factors in the injury-coping relationship exists. It has been suggested, for example, that the nature of the sport, starting status of the athlete, age of the athlete, and the coach's leadership style may influence the response and recovery to sport injury.[3,23] Petitpas and Danish[28] also argued that the overt visibility of a sport injury may effect an athlete's response and subsequent coping mechanisms. Most of these factors have received limited attention in the literature so that their exact role in the coping response and recovery from sport injury is uncertain. To date, there is a paucity of research that has examined the influence of cultural variability on the choice and effect of different coping strategies. Further investigation into the effects of these variables on coping behaviour following a sport injury and subsequent recovery process is needed.

Conclusions

In 1978, Pearlin and Schooler[57] asserted that no coping strategy would work for every individual in every situation, and this observation holds true today.[1] With the significant variability among individuals and across situations, there is no normative pattern with respect to coping. Each person faces a particular set of circumstances within the context of a unique personal history. Despite rigorous studies that have attempted to understand the role of coping in the stress process and the relationships between various coping strategies and outcomes, we still face many unanswered questions about the coping process. As Pearlin[35] suggested, we need to expand our research beyond an explanation of how individuals cope, to the conditions under which coping effectiveness is enhanced. Moreover, Madden[58] indicated that fruitful areas for future research are the types of strategies used, the effectiveness of these strategies, and how these strategies change over time.

In the process of studying ways in which athletes cope with injury, medical practitioners need to consider factors such as the stressors experienced by the athlete, the meaning and value for identity development that the injury has for the athlete, as well as personal and contextual factors that influence the coping process. By doing so, medical practitioners and sport psychologists would have a clearer understanding of the forces affecting the adjustment to injury and a better account for the fact that athletes experiencing the same stressor of injury are affected differently.

An implicit assumption exists that coping strategies are effective or ineffective depending on whether they enhance mastery over the environment or improve the person–environment relationship. In this way, 'coping is viewed as tantamount to solving problems...' (see ref. 6, p. 138 therein). While problem-solving is desirable, not all stressors are amenable to being solved. Furthermore, this view is limiting as there are many other positive developmental outcomes associated with coping. The case of an injured athlete is an excellent example. A career-ending injury cannot be 'fixed' or 'solved', but the athlete may grow in other substantial ways by coping with the injury. He/she may learn more about personal and situational resources available, his/her identity without sport, and may develop a sense of competence and efficacy in dealing with life's challenges. This athlete may learn skills to facilitate coping with future inevitable stressors. An emphasis on problem-solving also devalues other objectives of coping, such as the maintenance of self-esteem or a positive outlook in the face of unchangeable situations.

Research consistently supports the use of multiple coping strategies or having a versatile repertoire of coping strategies for healthy adjustment to life's demands[6,9] and athletic injury.[3] In other words, athletes will fare better with the adjustment of injury and other life stressors if they have at their disposal a range of emotion-focused and problem-focused coping strategies. Sport provides a unique opportunity to develop coping skills in young people. Inherent in sport, are experiences of injury, frustration, disappointment, challenge, and personal growth, with which the athlete needs to learn to cope. Medical practitioners and other support people may assist an athlete cope with injury; specifically, by considering the individual characteristics of the athlete, the meaning of the injury for the athlete, the nature of the injury (including the type, severity, timing, etc.), and the context in which the athlete trains and works. With an athlete-centred system and the appropriate supports from coaches, parents, and healthcare providers, athletes may develop important coping skills for sport and other facets of life.

References

1. Aldwin, C. (1994). *Stress, coping and development. An integrative perspective.* Guilford, New York.
2. Crossman, J., Gluck, L., and Jamieson, J. (1995). The emotional responses of injured athletes. *New England Journal of Sports Medicine*, **23**, 1–2.
3. Brewer, B., Linder, D., and Phelps, C. (1995). Situational correlates of emotional adjustment to athletic injury. *Clinical Journal of Sport Medicine*, **5**, 241–45.
4. Smith, A. (1996). Psychological impact of injuries in athletes. *Sports Medicine*, **22**, 391–405.
5. Fleming, R., Baum, A., and Singer, J. (1984). Toward an integrative approach to the study of stress. *Journal of Personality and Social Psychology*, **46**, 939–49.
6. Lazarus, R. and Folkman, S. (1984). *Stress, appraisal and coping.* Springer, New York.
7. White, R. (1974). Strategies of adaptation: An attempt at systematic description. In *Coping and adaptation* (ed. V. Coelho, D. Hamburg, and J. Adams), pp. 47–68. Basic Books, New York.
8. Pearlin, L. and Aneshensel, C. (1986). Coping and social supports: Their functions and applications. In *Applications of social science to clinical medicine and health* (ed. L. Aiken and D. Mechanic), pp. 53–74. Rutgers University Press, New Jersey.
9. Wethington, E. and Kessler, R. (1991). Situations and processes of coping. In *The social context of coping* (ed. J. Eckenrode), pp. 13–29. Plenum Press, New York.
10. Stone, A. and Neale, J. (1984). New measures of daily coping: development and preliminary results. *Journal of Personality and Social Psychology*, **46**, 892–906.
11. Folkman, S. (1984). Personal control and stress and coping processes: a theoretical analysis. *Journal of Personality and Social Psychology*, **46**, 839–52.
12. Folkman, S. and Lazarus, R. (1988). *The ways of coping questionnaire.* Consulting Psychologists Press, Palo Alto, CA.
13. Kaplan, H. (1996). *Psychosocial stress. Perspectives on structure, theory, life course and methods.* Academic Press, New York.
14. Vitaliano, P., DeWolfe, D., Maiuro, R., Russo, R., and Katon, W. (1990). Appraised changeability of a stressor as a modifier of the relationship between coping and depression. *Journal of Personality and Social Psychology*, **59**, 582–92.
15. Cutrona, C. and Russell, D. (1990). Type of social support and specific stress: Toward a theory of optimal matching. In *Social support: an interactional view* (ed. G. Sarason, B. Sarason, and G. Pierce), pp. 319–66. Wiley, New York.
16. Taylor, S. and Aspinwall, L. (1996). Mediating and moderating processes in psychosocial stress. In *Psychosocial stress* (ed. H. Kaplan), pp. 85–110. Academic Press, New York.

17. Forsythe, C. and Compas, B. (1987). Interaction of cognitive appraisals of stressful events and coping: Testing the goodness of fit hypothesis. *Cognitive Therapy and Research*, **11**, 473–85.
18. Anderson, M. and Williams, J. (1988). A model of stress and athletic injury: Prediction and prevention. *Journal of Sport and Exercise Psychology*, **10**, 296–306.
19. Heil, J. (1993). *Psychology of sport injury*. Human Kinetics, Champaign, IL.
20. Wiese-Bjornstal, D. and Smith, A. (1993). Counseling strategies for enhanced recovery of injured athletes within a team approach. In *Psychological bases of sport injuries* (ed. D. Pargman), pp. 149–82. Fitness Information Technology, Morgantown, WV.
21. Holahan, C. and Moos, R. (1990). Life stressors, resistance factors, and improved psychological functioning: An extension of the stress resistance paradigm. *Journal of Personality and Social Psychology*, **58**, 909–17.
22. Pearlin, L., Lieberman, M., Menaghan, E., and Mullen, J. (1981). The stress process. *Journal of Health and Social Behavior*, **22**, 337–56.
23. Flint, F. (1998). Integrating sport psychology and sports medicine in research: the dilemmas. *Journal of Applied Sport Psychology*, **10**, 83–102.
24. Grove, J. R. and Gordon, A. M. D. (1995). The psychological aspects of injury in sport. In *Science and medicine in sport* (2nd edn) (ed. J. Bloomfield et al.), pp. 194–205. Blackwell, Cambridge.
25. Grove, J., Hanrahan, S., and Stewart, R. (1990). Attributions for rapid or slow recovery from sports injuries. *Canadian Journal of Sport Sciences*, **15**, 107–14.
26. Laubach, W., Brewer, B., Van Raalte, J., and Petitpas, A. (1996). Attributions for recovery and adherence to sport injury rehabilitation. *Australian Journal of Science and Medicine in Sport*, **28**, 30–4.
27. Wasley, D. and Lox, C. L. (1998). Self-esteem and coping responses in athletes with acute versus chronic injuries. *Perceptual and Motor Skills*, **86**, 1402.
28. Petitpas, A. and Danish, S. J. (1995). Caring for injured athletes. In *Sport psychology intervention* (ed. S. M. Murphy), pp. 255–81. Human Kinetics, Champaign, IL.
29. Smith, A., Scott, S., O'Fallon, W., and Young, M. (1990). The emotional responses of athletes to injury. *Mayo Clinic Proceedings*, **65**, 38–50.
30. Smith, A., Stuart, M., Wiese-Bjornstal, D., Milliner, E., O'Fallon, W, and Crowson, C. (1993). Competitive athletes; pre and post injury mood state and self-esteem. *Mayo Clinic Proceedings*, **68**, 939–47.
31. Wiese-Bjornstal, D., Smith, A., and LaMott, E. (1995). A model of psychologic response to athletic injury and rehabilitation. *Athletic Training: Sports Health Care Perspective*, **1**, 17–30.
32. Terry, D. (1994). Determinants of coping: The role of stable and situational factors. *Journal of Personality and Social Psychology*, **66**, 895–910.
33. Rutter, M. (1991). Psychological resilience and protective mechanisms. In *Risk and protective factors in the development of psychopathology* (ed. D. Cicchetti, K. Nuechterlien, and S. Weintraub), pp. 181–214. Cambridge University Press, New York.

34. Kleiber, D., Greendorfer, S., Blinde, E., and Samdahl, D. (1987). Quality of exit from university sports and subsequent life satisfaction. *Sociology of Sport Journal*, **4**, 28–36.
35. Pearlin, L. (1991). The study of coping. An overview of problems and directions. In *The social context of coping* (ed. J. Eckenrode), pp. 261–76. Plenum Press, New York.
36. Gould, D., Udry, E., Bridges, D., and Beck, L. (1997). How to help elite athletes cope psychologically with season-ending injuries. *Athletic Therapy Today*, **2**, 50–3.
37. Quinn, A. and Fallon, B. (1999). The changes in psychological characteristics and reactions of elite athletes from injury onset until full recovery. *Journal of Applied Sport Psychology*, **11**, 210–29.
38. Stanton, A. and Snider, P. (1993). Coping with a breast cancer diagnosis: A prospective study. *Health Psychology*, **12**, 16–23.
39. Scheier, M. and Carver, C. (1992). Effects of optimism on psychological and physical well-being: Theoretical overview and empirical update. *Cognitive Therapy and Research*, **16**, 201–28.
40. Thoits, P. (1991). Gender differences in coping with emotional distress. In *The social context of coping* (ed. J. Eckenrode), pp. 107–33. Plenum Press, New York.
41. Gilligan, C. (1993). *In a different voice. Psychological theory and women's development*. Harvard University Press, Cambridge, MA.
42. Brewer, B. W. (1994). Review and critique of models of psychological adjustment to athletic injury. *Journal of Applied Sport Psychology*, **6**, 87–100.
43. Johnson, U. (1996). The multiply injured versus the first-time injured athlete during rehabilitation: a comparison of nonphysical characteristics. *Journal of Sport Rehabilitation*, **5**, 293–304.
44. Warner, M. and Amato, H. (1997). The mind: an essential healing tool for rehabilitation. *Athletic Therapy Today*, **2**, 37–41.
45. Haggerty, R., Sherrod, L., Garmezy, N., and Rutter, M. (1996). *Stress, risk, and resilience in children and adolescents*. Cambridge University Press, Cambridge.
46. Booth, A. and Amato, P. (1991). Divorce and psychological stress. *Journal of Health and Social Behavior*, **32**, 396–407.
47. Rosenfield, S. (1992). The costs of sharing: wives' employment and husbands' mental health. *Journal of Health and Social Behaviour*, **33**, 213–25.
48. Norris, F. and Murrell, S. (1984). Protective function of resources related to life events, global stress and depression in older adults. *Journal of Health and Social Behavior*, **25**, 424–37.
49. Hughes, R. and Coakley, J. (1991). Positive deviance among athletes: The implications of overconformity to the sport ethic. *Sociology of Sport Journal*, **8**, 307–25.
50. Nixon, H. (1992). A social network analysis of influences on athletes to play with pain and injuries. *Journal of Sport and Social Issues*, **16**, 127–35.

51. Nixon, H. (1993). Accepting the risks of pain and injury in sport: Mediated cultural influences on playing hurt. *Sociology of Sport Journal*, **10**, 183–96.
52. Nixon, H. (1994). Coaches' views of risk, pain, and injury in sport, with special reference to gender differences. *Sociology of Sport Journal*, **11**, 79–87.
53. Nixon, H. (1994). Social pressure, social support, and help seeking for pain and injuries in college sports networks. *Journal of Sport and Social Issues*, **18**, 340–55.
54. Nixon, H. (1996). Explaining pain and injury attitudes and experiences in sport in terms of gender, race, and sports status factors. *Journal of Sport and Social Issues*, **20**, 33–44.
55. Young, K. and White, P. (1995). Sport, physical danger, and injury: The experiences of elite women athletes. *Journal of Sport and Social Issues*, **19**, 45–61.
56. Young, K., White, P., and McTeer, W. (1994). Body talk: Male athletes reflect on sport, injury, and pain. *Sociology of Sport Journal*, **11**, 175–94.
57. Pearlin, L. and Schooler, C. (1978). The structure of coping. *Journal of Health and Social Behavior*, **19**, 2–21.
58. Madden, C. (1995). Ways of coping. In *Sports psychology: Theory, applications and issues* (ed. T Morris and J. Summers), pp. 288–310. Wiley, New York.

6   *Creating an environment for recovery*

Adrian Taylor and Caroline Marlow

Adherence to what: Defining the behavior?

We know a great deal about adherence levels to fitness and exercise programs, and adoption and maintenance of a wide range of health-promoting
behaviors. There is relatively less evidence about how good athletes are at
adhering to a program of rehabilitation following a sports injury. However,
the few studies that have examined this show that adherence rates may vary
considerably depending on the setting, medical history, severity of the injury,
stage of season, importance attached to (or level of) sports participation, and
many other factors. Perhaps the most critical factor though is whether the
rehabilitation program is to take place independently at home or in a supervised facility. Evidence suggests that adherence may be considerably higher
in a supervised setting[1, 2] or in sporting cultures which are supportive of the
recovering athlete.

The most fundamental question within adherence to injury rehabilitation
is adherence to what? There are often many components to a rehabilitation
program, all of which, we believe, require athlete commitment and adherence if the chances of recovery are to be optimized. For example, the athlete should attend all scheduled meetings with the therapist either at the
clinic or the gymnasium. Similarly, the athlete should complete home-based
exercises to the recommended intensity, frequency, and duration. Several
researchers have developed questionnaires to monitor adherence to different facets of the rehabilitation program.[3, 4] As a medical practitioner, you
will obviously keep medical records, but are they detailed enough to monitor levels of adherence to all components of the rehabilitation program?
Other chapters in this book focus on behaviors associated with optimizing
recovery, such as various aspects of psychological skills training. This
chapter is concerned with adherence to both physical and psychological
skills training that may enhance the rehabilitation process. The chapter
may therefore also be applicable to enhancing adherence to psychological
skills training.

Why is adherence to your prescribed rehabilitation program important?
Few studies have examined the dose-response relationship between rehabili-

tation and the rate of recovery from sports injuries, but we must assume that there is an optimal amount of whatever is recommended to ensure the most rapid recovery. Of course, trial and error may be necessary in some circumstances, but generally we employ a principle of 'evidence-based' practice. It is important to recognize that doing too much is also an adherence problem, which can mean failing to take the appropriate rest, or doing more of a specific exercise than was prescribed.

The main reason for monitoring adherence is to know what is working and what isn't. Without knowing what an athlete is doing when away from a supervised session it will be impossible to:

(1) attribute the rate of recovery to any specific element of the program, and modify programs accordingly;

(2) be a truly reflective medical practitioner who is able to offer the most beneficial rehabilitation programs for the athlete;

(3) know how well an athlete is coping with the injury and rehabilitation—levels of adherence (and motivation to engage in the rehabilitation program) may provide an indication of the emotional response and stage of emotional rehabilitation;

(4) know whether further motivational strategies are needed to support the athlete in their rehabilitation program;

(5) identify any behaviors that are counterproductive to the rehabilitation process.

Determinants of adherence

If adherence rates vary so much, what do we know about the factors or determinants of adherence to sport injury rehabilitation programs? There are a number of studies that have focused on this question,[2, 5–9] but we can also draw upon the large field of literature concerned with adherence to exercise programs in general and many other health behaviors.[10]

One way to examine the many different factors is to divide them into three categories. We prefer the following classification system. First, those factors that are concerned with the athlete's own perceptions, values, and attitudes towards the rehabilitation behavior in question, and also the intended outcomes from that rehabilitation program. We will call these 'predisposing factors'. Second, those factors that determine the impact of the interactions between the athlete and the medical practitioner, coach, and other important individuals on adherence. These will be referred to as 'reinforcing factors'. Third, the way in which the environment and nature of the rehabilitation program is established and modified, called 'enabling factors'.

Attitudes, beliefs, knowledge, values, emotions, and intentions (predisposing factors)

Other chapters in this book have examined the emotional responses of an injured athlete so we will not dwell on this for long. When an athlete arrives for treatment of an acute injury this may be the most obvious course of action due to the disabling nature of the injury. However, emotions do influence the decision to seek medical assistance for chronic injuries and they also affect the level of adherence to any prescribed treatment for both acute and chronic injuries.

How important is it for an athlete to understand and have knowledge about the cause and the diagnosis and prognosis of an injury? Should we spend time explaining the anatomic underpinnings of an injury using 3-dimensional models? There is no empirical evidence that says 'Yes', but intuitively there would seem to be a lot of support for spending time on this for three reasons. First, athletes, like any other patient, respond well to feeling that their injury is unique and personal. Second, understanding the process of injury helps an athlete to appreciate why certain rehabilitation techniques are required and, in turn, why time and commitment to the rehabilitation program is needed to promote healing. Third, it gives the athlete a sense of control and reduces worry that harm is being done, particularly during a rehabilitation program that may involve pain.

An athlete's level of knowledge and understanding (not necessarily of technical terms and jargon) will often be the basis for appropriate beliefs about rehabilitation behaviors and associated outcomes. We say 'will often' because it is sometimes surprising to hear quite knowledgeable athletes express beliefs about the value of including something in a rehabilitation program for which there is no rationale or evidence, but they have associated its efficacy on the basis of vicarious experience. For example, a friend may have had a 'similar injury' and recovered very quickly without taking rest, even though knowledge suggests that this would be counterproductive. The theoretical link between knowledge, beliefs, attitudes, intentions to do something, and actual rehabilitation behaviors is shown in Fig. 6.1. Beliefs are seen as specific thoughts about positive and negative outcomes associated with a behavior, whereas attitudes are generalized favorable or less-favorable thoughts about behaviors, objects, or concepts.[11] Thus, a (positive or negative) attitude towards a new rehabilitation program is generated from the sum of negative and positive beliefs about the potential value of that program. This will be important when we look at changing cognitions to enhance adherence later in this chapter.

Intentions to behave are not only dependent on an individual's personal beliefs and attitudes, but also upon the perceived beliefs and attitudes of important others. The general cognition about injury, rehabilitation behavior, and associated outcome expectations within a sports rehabilitation set-

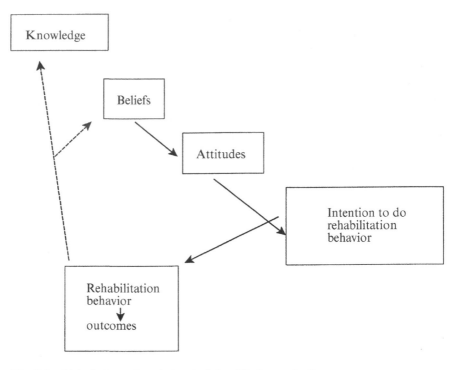

Fig. 6.1   Links between knowledge, beliefs, attitudes, and adherence.

ting may therefore influence the way individuals behave. This chapter is about enhancing adherence through the use of strategies for individuals, but it does not lose sight of the fact that the motivational climate or environment must be right.

Interactions with therapist, coach, parent, and other players (reinforcing factors)

Following on from the previous section, important others, such as a coach, teacher, parent, and other players, reinforce the value of specific rehabilitation behaviors. The medical practitioner has, of course, the potential to be highly influential.[10, 12–15] When the rehabilitation program is to be undertaken by the athlete without supervision, then understanding the components of the regimen and how they are to be conducted in terms of frequency and duration is fundamental to the athlete adhering to the program or not. In one unique study, athletes were interviewed immediately after leaving the consultation with a medical practitioner.[16] Only 23% could fully describe their program accurately and 23% did not know why they had to do what had been prescribed. Interestingly, all the athletes believed that they did understand what to do. Communication skills and processes, involving many medical practitioners, have been widely examined in the health psychology literature. One may assume that athletes will take a greater interest in, and have a greater awareness of, their bodies than non-athletes, thereby enhancing the communication process. However, as indicated in the study above,[16] this may be a dangerous assumption.

Evidence has been found of a self-fulfilling prophecy in the sports injury context.[17, 18] Within the medical practitioner–patient interaction, there may be a danger that through verbal and non-verbal communication the medical practitioner distinguishes between those most and least likely to follow a rehabilitation program. As such, if the medical practitioner's adherence expectations of the athlete are low, the self-fulfilling prophecy suggests that the nature of the prescribed exercises and the effort needed to motivate the athlete will be lower, and, sure enough, lower levels of adherence follow.

Levels of motivation to adhere to a rehabilitation program may also be dependent on the degree of satisfaction an athlete derives from a consultation. The topic of patient satisfaction has also been widely examined in the health psychology literature.[12,13] Two studies have measured athlete satisfaction using the Sports Injury Clinic Athlete Satisfaction Scale (SICASS).[19, 20] It included three dimensions, namely: perceived empathy, communication skills, and technical competence. It appeared that athletes were more critical of the empathy shown, perhaps because they felt in a better position to judge this dimension than the other aspects, or indeed the medical practitioners really did not, or did not try, to understand the true implications of the injury for the athlete. Surprisingly though, the researchers failed to find a relationship between the level of satisfaction and subsequent adherence to the rehabilitation program.[21]

The environment, stimulus, and reinforcement control (enabling factors)

The provision for sports injury treatment and rehabilitation varies enormously around the world, and may be dependent on the type of sport and the sports setting. For example, a team athlete may have access to a network of medical support, whereas an individual athlete may be relatively isolated. Also, athletes competing in interscholastic and intercollegiate sport or in professional sport in North America may have access to much better provision than other athletes. Athletic training rooms and designated sports injury centers can provide excellent on-site facilities to provide the stimulus and reinforcement to enable athletes to engage in rehabilitation programs. We say 'may' because environments are not just physical buildings but they also involve athlete perceptions and interpretation. Psychologists talk about changing motivational climates (environments). Within the same building, one study observed different motivational climates from one group of athletes to another.[22] For example, one group of team players quickly engaged in comparisons with others, whereas other groups, including skiers, jockeys, and other individual sport athletes, adopted more individualized goals. On occasion, a climate allowing interathlete competition to take place in all facets of the program was found to lead to a sense of failure or retarded progress. The use of self-referenced goals was thus recommended.

Within this section, it is important to consider the possible impact of environments which are not enabling for athletes. Both the quantity and quality of social support is important. Without regular access to emotional and instrumental (including information, medical guidance, and technical advice) support, the rehabilitation process may slow down or involve avoidable complications. We will say more about improving enabling factors for both facility and home-based programs.

Strategies to increase adherence

Changing predisposing factors

Information—knowledge

How often in the early parts of an initial consultation do you include attempts to find out what an athlete knows about an injury, beyond asking if it is recurrent? Do you engage with the athlete as someone who can educate you, and someone who has a wealth of knowledge about how the injury occurred, how it feels, and what would be most likely to work as a rehabilitation program? The secret for the medical practitioner who wants to increase the likelihood of rehabilitation behaviors being adopted and maintained, is to extract as much verbal and non-verbal information from the athlete as possible—and to be seen to act upon it. Every athlete has a level of understanding about an injury. If the medical practitioner can quickly determine that level, then the consultation can take place without fear of being seen to ignore the athlete, or of being condescending, and the athlete can be challenged to be a part of the alliance in setting a rehabilitation program. Consultations in which there is a clear dominant (medical practitioner)–submissive (athlete) relationship are likely to lead to lower levels of adherence. A valuable strategy might be to use the injury as an opportunity for the athlete to learn about his/her body and the effects of training and rehabilitation.

Counseling—attitudes, values, matched stage of change approaches

Earlier we discussed the nature of the relationship between the medical practitioner and the patient. It is easy to expect or assume that athletes want to be prescribed a rehabilitation program and will automatically follow this to the letter. That may well not be the case. The challenge then is to motivate athletes to adopt and maintain rehabilitation behaviors (including appropriate rest). The medical practitioner takes on the role of counselor and/or psychologist in these circumstances. One approach to counseling is through motivational interviewing[14] in which the client is encouraged to present the ideas for change themselves through counselor-led discussions. Those discussions may use the 'Stages of Change' framework[23] (see Table 6.1) as a basis for moving clients from never having thought about a behavior (precontemplation) to maintaining it.

Since this model (Table 6.1) was proposed, it has been widely applied to changing many different behaviors, including exercise for health.[24] It has not, to our knowledge, previously been proposed for use in the sports injury setting, but let's examine where it holds potential. If you are trying to increase stretching behavior, for example, as part of a rehabilitation program, it would be initially important to identify where someone lies on the continuum (or even circle, since passing from stage to stage sometimes occurs in a cyclical manner). When the athlete's position has been established it becomes possible to counsel him/her towards appropriate cognitive and behavioral techniques. Table 6.2 demonstrates how counseling strategies are clearly matched with the stage of readiness to adopt or maintain a particular behavior. As we identified initially, it must be remembered that a rehabilitation program may involve a wide variety of different behaviors. An injured athlete may be at different stages for each one, so the counseling role should relate to this stage for maximum effectiveness.

There are other ways of approaching behavior change and adherence. An understanding of a number of cognitive and behavioral approaches may help you to be more effective in motivating or encouraging athletes to adopt and maintain rehabilitation behaviors.[25] The Stages of Change model does not replace the need to understand more conventional models used to change behavior, although ideally models can be used in combination.

Earlier we identified a simplified link between knowledge, beliefs, attitudes, intentions, and behavior (Fig. 6.1). To combine this with the Stages of Change, we can see that knowledge, beliefs, attitudes, and intentions all have the potential to alter throughout time, and thus affect the athlete's position

Table 6.1 Stages of change for adoption and maintenance of sports injury rehabilitation behaviors

Stage 1	Precontemplation
Stage 2	Contemplation
Stage 3	Preparation
Stage 4	Action
Stage 5	Maintaining

Table 6.2 Matching stage of readiness to change with counseling strategy

Stage	Strategy	Counselor action
Precontemplation	Cognitive	Try to raise doubts about inappropriate behavior (e.g. not enough stretching). Heighten athlete's perceived risk associated with inappropriate behavior.
	Behavioral	Suggest athlete talks to others and reads about appropriate behavior.
Contemplation	Cognitive	Encourage athlete to state perceived benefits of behavior change. Heighten athlete's perceived risk associated with inappropriate behavior. Increase athlete's self-efficacy (beliefs that they can change behavior).
	Behavioral	Suggest athlete gains further information about changing behavior.
Preparation	Cognitive	Discuss options associated with behavior change (e.g., expectations, goals, choices, etc.) and plan steps to change (e.g., when, how, what). Increase athlete's self-efficacy that they can complete steps to change.
	Behavioral	Find a partner to do new behavior with. Enlist social support (people to prompt, encourage, reinforce, etc.). Look for other behaviors to substitute with new one.
Action	Cognitive	Emphasize feelings (e.g., less effort, more flexibility, stronger), and encourage greater perceived control over rehabilitation progress.
	Behavioral	Encourage self-rewarding strategies and use of others for support. Encourage athlete to commit self to the rehabilitation with continual self-talk and reminders to do it.
Maintenance	Cognitive	Discuss relapse prevention strategies. Emphasize goal attainments and link action with benefits.
	Behavioral	Add new activities, and help others in their rehabilitation program. Use stimulus and reinforcement control strategies (see below).

within the Stages of Change framework. To change behavior or to maximize adherence we would therefore suggest using strategies that challenge and change those athlete's beliefs and attitudes that are presently preventing the completion of rehabilitation behaviors. One such technique is the decision-balance sheet (Table 6.3). This technique can be used to aid progression through all the identified stages, but it is a particularly useful tool for those athletes who are in the precontemplation-to-preparation stages or are having problems achieving maintenance. We have found the following steps useful:

1. Select a specific behavior (including rest or restricted activity) that may be critical to the rehabilitation program and which may be at risk of non-adherence.

2. Encourage the athlete to identify the perceived gains and losses to him or herself and others, and how the new behavior might bring approval from themselves or others.

3. Explore with the athlete any other potential gains, and highlight the identified gains. Discuss the potential losses and get the athlete to review these with the aim of removing them as barriers/losses.

4. Review all gains and losses and highlight the potential gains and losses of adopting or maintaining the rehabilitation behavior.

The decision-balance sheet (see Table 6.3) is a technique that has been successfully used in the exercise setting to increase adherence.[26] Simply identifying the gains and losses appears to clarify for the individual just what may be involved in the behavior of interest, and provides an opportunity to emphasize the positive aspects and minimize the negative consequences. Sometimes, such beliefs may be quite different from what may be expected. For example, some athletes relish the opportunity to participate with pain and injury within a complex social network of values.[27]

More specific beliefs may also be the target. The value of raising fear about the negative consequences of behaving in a certain way has been examined through the Health Belief Model[28] across many different preventive health behaviors. Here we are interested in the following question: 'Is adherence increased by suggesting to an athlete that full recovery may never be achieved if a rehabilitation program is not adhered to, or that full recovery will be seriously delayed by non-adherence?'

Perhaps, as a medical practitioner, you have used this approach to motivate athletes. The literature is very sparse, but one study has suggested that those with lower perceptions of the severity and seriousness of a sports injury were less likely to adhere to a home-based rehabilitation program than those with a greater perceived threat.[2] There are two implications of this for the medical practitioner. First, you can ascertain from the athlete the perceptions of threat and fear associated with the injury; and, second, you can seek to

Table 6.3 Decision-balance sheet for use with injured athletes

	Gains	Losses
Self		
Important others		
Self-approval		
Approval by others		

raise fear about the consequences of not completing the rehabilitation program. As a word of caution, further research evidence is needed to fully support the latter course, as in other situations where fear has been used to promote behavior change the evidence is unconvincing.

Another athlete perception that is critical to assess when providing a rehabilitation program, is whether the athlete actually feels capable of performing its various components, and whether each component is seen to be of any value for recovery. Self-efficacy and outcome expectations are perhaps the most predictive of subsequent behavior, across many different settings. In the rehabilitation setting, if you as a medical practitioner are to ask any questions to determine if an athlete will adhere to a program, it will be:

1.   Do you feel that you will be able to ...?

2.   How do you feel that doing ... will benefit your speed of recovery?

To avoid the likely response of a simple 'yes' from the first question you should append additional phrases such as:

Do you feel that you will be able to ...?

   '... even when you have other things to do?'

   '... even when it gives you pain?'

   '... even when others offer no support?'

These questions can then, in turn, be probed for further information.

Asking about perceived capabilities and expectations is the first step. The second step is to change these perceptions in a way that will increase the likelihood of adherence. The literature suggests that self-efficacy, the belief in perceived capability to perform a specific behavior, comes from four key sources:[29]

(1)   performance attainment;

(2)   verbal and social persuasion;

(3)   imitation and modeling;

(4)   judgments of physiological states.

Performance attainment

Injury rehabilitation programs are often unique in that the behavior(s) being recommended has never been performed before. If this is the case, then it may be difficult for an athlete to estimate whether some specific exercises can be performed. If you are giving an athlete a number of home-based exercises to do, you may routinely ask them to go through the rehabilitation program with you in the clinic, thereby demonstrating an ability to perform them and enhancing performance attainment. This is fine if the source of low self-efficacy is due to perceptions of physical immobility. If the perceived barriers are time or lack of support, then you will need to enhance perceptions of performance attainment through eliciting examples of when the athlete has overcome such obstacles, perhaps to accomplish other tasks. The decision balance sheet is also particularly useful for reviewing time priorities.

Verbal and social persuasion

No matter what you say to encourage adherence (not forgetting that this may also include reducing normal training and competition), it may have little effect. Perhaps the key thing is that the same message comes from a number of sources, particularly from those with whom the athlete has regular contact. If, in an athletic training room, there is generally a low work ethos among injured athletes, or poor adherence, it will be critical to change this whole climate to increase self-efficacy. Enlisting others for support and to prompt rehabilitation behaviors is something that appeared in Table 6.2.

Imitation and modeling

When doubt about being able to adhere to a particular regimen is expressed, then one commonly used strategy is to recall how other well-known athletes have overcome the same problems. Demonstrating how specific exercises should be performed in the clinic or training room is, of course, normal practice. Identifying a buddy to train with can be a highly effective way of increasing self-efficacy, both as a support and as a role model if the buddy has experienced a similar injury. A new technological approach is also presently being tested and would appear to have some value for home-based programs. In this case, fairly standard exercises for athletes with an anterior cruciate ligament injury are being reproduced on a videotape, with the prescribed type, number of repetitions, and sets shown for each individual athlete. The athlete takes the video home and follows the program in the comfort of his/her own home, or potentially in a gym.

Judgments of physiological states

One of the key doubts about performing rehabilitation exercises is that they induce pain, and so a level of tolerance is required. For the athlete, pain may raise fears that the injury is being aggravated. Dealing with pain in a rehabilitation program is quite different from playing through in competition, when physiological arousal is high and sport is distracting. Giving an athlete the confidence to know how much pain to endure and how to endure it is not easy. Going through the exercises in the clinic is one obvious strategy, and this can be done in conjunction with several pain management strategies. If an athlete feels more capable of dealing with pain, then this will affect their self-efficacy to perform some of the more painful exercises. Adherence to rest or reduced involvement in sport may also be problematic. If you recommend several weeks of inactivity then an athlete may immediately think that this advice is difficult to follow due to personal dependence on being physically active, and the physical and psychological feelings associated with that. You may well want to recommend alternative forms of exercise which are not restricted by the injury.

Summary

In summary, the following strategies are closely linked to increasing perceptions of self-efficacy:

1. Provide time for the athlete to go through the specific components to confirm understanding, but more importantly to provide the athlete with a belief that they can, for example, perform the exercise or stretch, or restrict activity.

2. Use role models as examples of how others have performed a rehabilitation program.

3. Ask the athlete to recall examples of where specific forms of training (or rehabilitation) have been completed successfully and verbally attribute this to his or her own efforts.

4. Break the rehabilitation program into specific behaviors and set goals for each one.

5. Quickly identify the key potential stumbling blocks and focus on increasing self-efficacy for those specific actions.

Goal-setting

Providing athletes with goals is something medical practitioners use as part of their normal practice. But, how goal-setting is used by the medical practitioner varies considerably and may be different from the methods employed by a sports psychologist.[30] The idea that goals should be SMARTER (i.e. specific, measurable, attainable, realistic, time-based, evaluated, and recorded) is commonly accepted, as is the understanding and use of short- and long-term goals. However, less recognition and differentiation of process and outcome goals was reported among medical practitioners.[30]

Process goals are concerned with completing the rehabilitation program (despite the obstacles identified above), whereas outcome goals are about the level of functioning, on micro- (e.g., an ability to show a range of movement in a limb) and macro- (e.g., return to previous performance level) scales. The danger with an exclusive focus on outcome goals is that rehabilitation progress can be so case-specific. If progress is not achieved, then an athlete can be left with a sense of failure and even learned helplessness. If psychological rehabilitation is also recognized as important, then programs that lead to learned helplessness or a sense of failure should be avoided, particularly during the early phases of emotional response prior to acceptance. This is particularly pertinent for highly competitive athletes.

In one rehabilitation setting, athletes naturally sought to compete with fellow injured athletes on simple rehabilitation exercises involving resistance work, sometimes to the detriment of their progress.[30] An exclusive focus on outcome goals appeared to be linked to the perception that more weight lifted, more often, would not only enhance social acceptance, but also speed up rehabilitation rates.

On the other hand, injury provides an opportunity for athletes to develop new personal skills and a sense of achievement or mastery, at a time when life may take on a very different meaning from the one to which an athlete is accustomed.[31, 32]

There are five key principles of a task-oriented, goal-setting strategy:[32]

1. Help the athlete develop management skills that are transferable between rehabilitation situations.
2. Help the athlete to establish rehabilitation schedules.
3. Provide opportunities for self-evaluation and self-monitoring.
4. Involve the athlete in decision-making.
5. Ensure individual progress is self-referenced.

The idea of a life development intervention, particularly for a long-term or serious injury that may be career-threatening, has been advocated elsewhere.[31] For such athletes, it is impossible to separate physical and psychological rehabilitation. The goal must be to work through the emotions associated with the injury to a point where 'acceptance' is reached.

Changing reinforcing factors

The nature and quality of interaction between the medical practitioner and athlete is also critical. The important questions to ask here are:

1. How do you appear to the athlete, and how does this influence adherence?
2. What do you typically do (through verbal and non-verbal communication style) that effects adherence?
3. What do you do with some athletes and not with others that is more likely to increase adherence?

Having observed many interactions between medical practitioners and athletes, one thing that really stands out as important for promoting athlete adherence is the natural empathetic nature of the medical practitioner. This can be achieved in two ways. First, by demonstrating a genuine interest in the athlete as an athlete (and not just a patient, as may occur in a general healthcare setting which is not sports-injury designated); and, second, by putting aside any personal medical agenda to reach a diagnosis, prognosis, and treatment plan in a way that encourages athlete-ownership of the problem.

Self-fulfilling prophecy

Earlier we wrote about the danger of the self-fulfilling prophecy. In a way, the effective medical practitioner must accept some responsibility for adherence, but how much? If an athlete appears unwilling to adhere to any prescribed regimen is that the athlete's choice or does the medical practitioner hold a 'duty-of-care' to maximize the likelihood of adherence: clearly, a medical philosophical issue. When a child goes to school, the parent(s) expect the teacher to try to motivate the child to learn rather than to dismiss him/her as uninterested. Likewise, when a coach sends an athlete to you, they expect you to not only offer technical expertise but also motivational empowerment. Evidence suggests that when a medical practitioner initially expected low levels of adherence, 75% of athletes (from self-report) did not subsequently adhere to recommended rest.[18] This compared with 32% who were initially expected to adhere. The question remains, was this due to the medical practitioner being particularly good at predicting who would or would not comply, or was it due to the self-fulfilling prophecy? In other words, through verbal and non-verbal communication early in the initial consultation, the medical practitioner picked up some clues that indicated the poor likelihood of subsequent adherence and hence took less effort to motivate the individual to adhere to the home-based treatment plan. Conversely, cues indicating a greater likelihood of adherence led to more effort by the medical practitioner to ensure adherence. You may well feel that you are consistent across all patients, but think of the times when you are tired or want to get away early for a pressing engagement.

If nothing else, after reading this section you may consciously view your interactions with athletes differently in the future. There may be four important implications here:

1. Reflect on the verbal and non-verbal cues you use to identify likely non-adherers.
2. Reflect on whether you see such athletes as a challenge or a turn-off.
3. Identify strategies you use to empower motivated and less-motivated athletes.
4. Attempt to use new strategies to empower less-motivated athletes.

Communication

We previously identified the poor communication of information as a cause of poor adherence. There is clearly a case for providing written instructions for standard rehabilitation exercises; yet, as one study reported,[16] these were only provided by 14% of the medical practitioners surveyed. We have already mentioned the idea of providing athletes with a take-home video that explicitly identifies what is expected, but this may be beyond the resources of most medical practitioners. In our experience, athletes typically want to know about their injury. If an athlete understands what caused an injury, and how preventive behaviors can reduce future risk, then such actions may follow. A working anatomical 3D model can be used to aid understanding of how specific rehabilitation exercises will impact on the injury. Providing reading material about the etiology and treatment of specific injuries, pitched at the right level, may also help to communicate technical information.

Creating athlete ownership of rehabilitation

Communicating information is important for not only pragmatic reasons, but also for empowerment. Engaging an athlete in the ownership of a rehabilitation program is likely to increase adherence. It is important to listen to athletes as educators and include them, whenever possible, in decision-making about the treatment plan. You can imagine two quite different approaches: in one case, the medical practitioner immediately steps into a white-coat-type dominating role and promptly goes through a mechanistic checklist of signs and symptoms before producing a diagnosis. In no time at all, a rehabilitation program has been offered and the athlete has barely said a word, but plays the submissive role superbly. In a second scenario, an athlete is given the opportunity to describe the signs and symptoms of the injury, previous injury history, level and personal meaning of involvement in sport, and knowledge of others who have had similar injuries and their prognosis and rehabilitation program. The mutual alliance (shared power) leads to an agreed rehabilitation program which suits the lifestyle of the athlete. Which do you think is more likely to enhance adherence?

Client satisfaction

We wrote earlier about athlete satisfaction in sports injury clinics. Although no relationship was found between levels of satisfaction and subsequent adherence to a rehabilitation program,[21] this link has been reported in other health psychology literature in different healthcare settings.[12] There is evidence that the nature of the relationship between medical practitioner and patient influences the levels of satisfaction and subsequent adherence to treatment. Not surprisingly, relationships involving respect, empathy, and sincerity, as well as communication skills, such as listening and the use of non-technical jargon or non-condescending language, are most likely to be associated with patient satisfaction.

How do you know if your athletes are satisfied? The Sports Injury Clinic Athlete Satisfaction Scale is shown in Appendix 2. You may want to add other aspects of satisfaction to it relating to cost, appointment waiting time, and other aspects of the service you provide. Be wary of biases in the way that people respond, as patient satisfaction is a rather emotive concept.[33] Patients do not want to bite the hand that feeds them. Another approach to understanding the nature of your relationships with athletes may be to ask a colleague to observe you and provide feedback, preferably in an open and non-threatening environment. You could also set up a video camera (with consent from your patients) and reflect on how your actions impact on the consultation.

Social support networks

Social support networks are important for injured athletes.[34] As a medical practitioner, information should be collected on both the amount and quality of support throughout the rehabilitation process, as this will help you to assess the athlete's support needs. Athletes are particularly liable to a lack of social support at this most needy time, as absence from the training environment often takes them away from their usual support networks and significant others. This is often particularly the case for athletes with long-term or career-ending injuries. Apart from taking the first step to identify potential problems with support networks, more proactive strategies can be employed. For example, links that have been made with the coach or training group can be used to encourage a support structure. Alternatively, the creation of buddy groups or partnerships enabling athletes with similar injuries, or with past experience of such injuries, to train together can be effective. Introductions or referrals to new training centers can also be invaluable.

Changing enabling factors

This final section is about providing the athlete with tools to aid motivation. Usually, the term 'behavioral modification' implies that one person is attempting to shape and modify the behavior of another through planned actions involving the presentation of stimuli and reinforcement schedules. Given the previous discussion about empowering athletes to take control of their own rehabilitation program, we do not wish to imply that behavior modification is being used to control athletes. Instead, we see the following section as one that you can use to give athletes greater control over their own rehabilitation behaviors.

Stimulus control

Stimulus control strategies are based on the principle that a prompt to do something will be more likely to trigger a desirable behavior than if no such cue was available. There are seven strategies listed below, which are supported within the exercise adherence literature, that you can use in your practice:[35]

1. Have the athlete set a regular time and/or setting to undertake the rehabilitation work. Time management is critical for doing anything, but it is worth remembering that when unable to be fully functional, the athlete suddenly has a lot of time available. Setting particular times for his/her rehabilitation training can help to provide the daily structure which an athlete is typically used to.

2. Ensure that the athlete engages in an adequate warm-up and initially avoids hard or more painful work in the rehabilitation session. When the next opportunity to work-out arises, enhance the athletes' motivation by encouraging them to think of the less-challenging parts of the session. Similarly, warming down and ending with something enjoyable may be less likely to leave the athlete with aversive thoughts and stimuli for the next session.

3. Gradually increase the athlete's rehabilitation targets. Again, if the athlete tries to do too much too soon it is likely to lead to poor long-term adherence.

4. The 'show-up' system. To help the athlete adhere to/remember a planned rehabilitation session, encourage them to put out their training clothes in a prominent place, perhaps the night before. Also encourage athletes to leave reminder notes and enlist a friend to provide prompts.

5. Sign a treatment plan agreement with the athlete and encourage him/her to display it in a prominent place to act as a prompt.

6. If the athlete knows that certain behaviors are likely to interfere with his/her rehabilitation program, encourage them to avoid conflicting influences.

7. Telephone or ask an important other person to phone the athlete to prompt completion of the rehabilitation program.

Reinforcement control

Reinforcement control strategies are based on the principle that a reward that follows a behavior is likely to increase the likelihood of that behavior being repeated when similar opportunities or stimuli are presented in the future. The ultimate reward for adherence to a rehabilitation program for an injured athlete is likely to be a return to competition. If short-term outcome goals are attained then this is likely to reinforce rehabilitation behavior. However, rehabilitation behaviors are only likely to become habitual if there are tangible or intangible rewards after each session, or, at least, on a regular basis. The strategies listed below have support in the exercise adherence literature,[35] and can be used within your practice.

1. Encourage the athlete to keep a rehabilitation diary and/or graph showing the process and outcome goal attainment. Get the athlete to read the diary regularly or display it in a prominent place to remind them of the progress made and to help them make the connection between doing something and real progress.

2. Encourage the athlete to award him/herself points for doing the rehabilitation work and to accumulate them to gain a tangible reward.

3. Encourage the athlete to enter into a contract with someone. The con-

tractor will provide a reward if the athlete demonstrates adherence to a rehabilitation program.

4. Teach the athlete to use visualization to experience the sensations of being able to achieve both short- and long-term goals and rewards.

5. If you provide a group rehabilitation setting, set up a lottery system in which each person contributes to a fund. All those who show complete adherence to their rehabilitation program are entered into the lottery for a winner to take the fund.

6. Premack principle:
   • help the athlete to select an enjoyable activity;
   • only allow the athlete to do that activity if the rehabilitation has been completed. Alternatively, encourage the athlete to do the rehabilitation while watching something they enjoy on TV.

7. Encourage the athlete to surround themselves with friends who offer encouragement and praise for achieving the process and outcome goals.

Summary

This chapter has been written as a practical guide to creating an environment for injury rehabilitation. An assumption is made that adherence is critical and that a rehabilitation program may involve many different components, requiring different degrees of support, athlete involvement and commitment, and time. Monitoring all these components by a medical practitioner may be impossible, but it is within the spirit of this chapter that the athlete will be given every opportunity to engage in this process. In addition, we acknowledge that the inclusion of many of these techniques will probably require you to commit more time to each athlete. However, we hope that you can see how this extra time could lead to a more successful application of your expertise, quicker and more successful athlete recovery, and greater athlete satisfaction.

A variety of factors that appear to be influential in achieving adherence have been considered under the headings: predisposing; reinforcing; and enabling factors. There will undoubtedly be overlap between these, but such a division provides a basis for you, the medical practitioner, to examine how you reflect on your own interactions with patients, and, hopefully, select new strategies which you will find useful and rewarding in your professional practice.

As psychologists, we do not have your technical skills. We have extensively observed professional practice in different cultures, and different treatment contexts, as both injured athletes and as sport psychologists. We hope that this chapter will enable you to view your work from a different perspective.

References

1. Fisher, A. C. (1990). Adherence to sports injury rehabilitation programmes. *Sports Medicine*, **9**, 151–8.
2. Taylor, A. H. and May, S. (1996). Threat and coping appraisal as determinants of compliance to sports injury rehabilitation: An application of protection motivation theory. *Journal of Sports Sciences*, **14**, 471–82.
3. May, S. and Taylor, A. H. (1994). The development and examination of various measures of patient compliance, for specific use with injured athletes. *Journal of Sports Science*, **12**, 180–181. [Abstract]
4. Brewer, B. W., Daly, J. M., Van Raalte, J. L., Petitpas, A. J., and Sklar, J. H. (1994). A psychometric evaluation of the rehabilitation adherence questionnaire. [Abstract]. Journal of Sport & Exercise Psychology, **16** (Suppl.), S34.
5. Brewer, B. W. (1999). Adherence to sport injury rehabilitation regimens. In *Adherence issues in sport and exercise* (ed. S. Bull), pp. 145–68. Wiley, Chichester.
6. Duda, J. L., Smart, A. E., and Tappe, M. K. (1989). Prediction of adherence in the rehabilitation of athletic injuries: An application of personal investment theory. *Journal of Sport and Exercise Psychology*, **11**, 367–81.
7. Fisher, A. C., Domm, M. A., and Wuest, D. A. (1988). Adherence to sports injury rehabilitation programs. *Physician and Sports Medicine*, **16**, 47–52.
8. Satterfield, M. J., Dowden, D., and Yasumura, K. (1990). Patient compliance for successful stress fracture rehabilitation. *Journal of Orthopaedic and Sports Physical Therapy*, **11**, 321–4.
9. Shaffer, S. M. (1992). Attributions and self-efficacy as predictors of rehabilitative success. Unpublished Master's thesis, University of Illinois at Urbana-Champaign.
10. Meichenbaum, D. and Turk, D. (1987). *Facilitating treatment adherence*. Plenum Press, New York.
11. Ajzen, I. and Fishbein, M. (1980). *Understanding attitudes and predicting social behavior*. Prentice Hall, Englewood Cliffs, NJ.
12. DiMatteo, M. R. and DiNicola, D. D. (1982). *Achieving patient compliance: the psychology of the medical practitioner's role*. Pergamon, Oxford.
13. Ley, P. (1988). *Communicating with patients: Improving communication, satisfaction and compliance*. Croom Helm, London.
14. Rollnick, S., Mason, P., and Butler, C. (1999). *Health behaviour change: A guide for practitioners*. Churchill Livingstone, London.
15. Weise, D. M. and Weiss, M. R. (1987). Psychological rehabilitation and physical injury: Implications for the sports medicine team. *The Sport Psychologist*, **1**, 318–30.
16. Webborn, A. D. J., Carbon, R. J., and Miller, B. (1997). Injury rehabilitation programs: What are we talking about? *Journal of Sport Rehabilitation*, **6**, 54–61.

17. Wilder, K. C. (1994). Clinicians' expectations and their impact on an athlete's compliance in rehabilitation. *Journal of Sport Rehabilitation*, **3**, 168–75.

18. Taylor, A. H. and May, S. (1995). Physiotherapists' expectations and their influence on compliance to sports injury rehabilitation. In *Proceedings of the IXth European Congress on Sports Psychology, Part 2* (ed. R. van Fraechem-Raway and Y. van den Auweele), pp. 619–25. Brussels, July 4–9, 1995.

19. May, S. (1995). An investigation into compliance with sports injury rehabilitation regimens. Unpublished doctoral dissertation, University of Brighton, UK.

20. Taylor, A. H. and May, S. (1995). Development of a sports injury clinic athlete satisfaction scale for auditing patients' perceptions. *Physiotherapy Theory and Practice*, **11**, 231–8.

21. Taylor, A. H. and May, S. (1997). *A prospective study of the relationship between patient satisfaction and sports injury rehabilitation compliance. Proceedings of the IXth World Congress of Sport Psychology*, Israel, July 5–9, 1997.

22. Gilbourne, D. (1998). Collaborative research involving the sport psychologist within sports injury settings: action research themes and processes. Unpublished doctoral dissertation, University of Brighton, UK.

23. Prochaska, J. O., DiClemente, C. C., and Norcross, J. C. (1992). In search of how people change. *American Psychologist*, **47**, 1102–14.

24. Reed, G. R. (1999). Adherence to exercise and the transtheoretical model of behavior change. In *Adherence issues in sport and exercise* (ed. S. Bull), pp. 19–46. Wiley, Chichester.

25. Worrel, T. W. (1992). The use of behavioural and cognitive techniques to facilitate achievement of rehabilitation goals. *Journal of Sport Rehabilitation*, **1**, 69–75.

26. Marcus, B., Rakowski, W., and Rossi, J. (1992). Assessing motivational readiness and decision making for exercise. *Health Psychology*, **11**, 257–61.

27. Nixon, H. L. (1992). A social network analysis of influences on athletes to play with pain and injuries. *Journal of Sport and Social Issues*, **16**, 127–35.

28. Janz, N. K. and Becker, M. H. (1984). The health belief model: A decade later. *Health Education Quarterly*, **11**, 1–47.

29. Bandura, A. (1977). *Social learning theory*. Prentice Hall, Englewood Cliffs, NJ.

30. Gilbourne, D., Taylor, A. H., Downie, G., and Newton, P. (1996). Goal setting during sports injury rehabilitation: A presentation of underlying theory, administration procedures and an athlete case study. *Sport, Exercise, Injury*, **2**, 192–201.

31. Danish, S. J., Petitpas, A. J., and Hale, B. D. (1993). Life development intervention for athletes: life skills through sports. *The Counselling Psychologist*, **21**, 352–85.

32. Gilbourne, D. and Taylor, A. H. (1998). From theory to practice: the integration of goal perspective theory and life development approaches within an injury-specific goal setting programme. *Journal of Applied Sports Psychology*, **10**, 124–39.

33. Rees Lewis, J. (1994). Patient views on quality care in general practice: literature review. *Social Science Medicine*, **39**, 655–70.
34. Udry, E. (1997). Coping and social support among injured athletes following surgery. *Journal of Sport & Exercise Psychology*, **19**, 71–90.
35. Leith, L. M. and Taylor, A. H. (1992). Behaviour modification and exercise adherence: A literature review. *Journal of Sport Behaviour*, **15**, 60–74.

Appendix A

The Sports Injury Rehabilitation Beliefs Survey (SIRBS)

The words 'rehabilitation program' should be read to mean any advice that you are given in order to assist the rehabilitation of your injury.

Please respond to the following statements using the scale shown below.

Very Strongly Disagree	Strongly Disagree	Disagree	Neither Agree nor Disagree	Agree	Strongly Agree	Very Strongly Agree
1	2	3	4	5	6	7

1. My recovery from injury may be hindered if I do not complete the rehabilitation program.

    1   2   3   4   5   6   7

2. In order to prevent a recurrence of this injury, my rehabilitation program is essential.

    1   2   3   4   5   6   7

3. The way to prevent my injury from worsening will be to follow my rehabilitation program.

    1   2   3   4   5   6   7

4. A successful and lasting recovery may not be possible if I do not complete my rehabilitation program.

    1   2   3   4   5   6   7

5. I am making it more likely that I will be re-injured by not doing what my rehabilitation involves.

    1   2   3   4   5   6   7

6. The rehabilitation program designed for me will ensure my complete recovery from this injury.

    1   2   3   4   5   6   7

7. Completion of my rehabilitate program will guarantee that I recover from my injury.

    1   2   3   4   5   6   7

8. Following the advice that I have been given will have a very large impact upon how quickly I will recover from my injury.

    1   2   3   4   5   6   7

9. I have absolute faith in the effectiveness of my rehabilitation program.

    1   2   3   4   5   6   7

10. I am very capable of successfully completing all aspects of my rehabilitation program, even if it involves being less active or something that may be discomforting.

    1   2   3   4   5   6   7

11. I consider myself able to stick with my rehabilitation program even though it may include activities that I do not enjoy.

    1   2   3   4   5   6   7

12. I will have no serious difficulty in following the instructions of my rehabilitation program.

    1   2   3   4   5   6   7

13. I believe that I will stick to my rehabilitation program despite any difficulties that I may encounter.

        1   2   3   4   5   6   7

14. Being fully recovered from injury is extremely important to me.

        1   2   3   4   5   6   7

15. As far as injuries go, mine is serious.

        1   2   3   4   5   6   7

16. I see this injury as a serious threat to my sport/exercise involvement.

        1   2   3   4   5   6   7

17. I fear that this injury will affect my long-term sports involvement.

        1   2   3   4   5   6   7

18. This injury is too serious to not follow medical advice.

        1   2   3   4   5   6   7

*19.Injuries like this are minor interruptions to my sport/exercise involvement.

        1   2   3   4   5   6   7

Items 1–5 deal with susceptibility
Items 6–9 deal with treatment efficacy
Items 10–13 deal with self-efficacy
Item 14 deals with rehabilitation value
Items 15–19 deal with severity
*Item reverse-coded

Reprinted with permission from Dr. Adrian Taylor.

Appendix B

Sports injury clinic athlete satisfaction scale

Write a number next to each statement indicating the extent to which you agree or disagree using the scale below.

Strongly disagree	Disagree	Neither agree nor disagree	Agree	Strongly agree
1	2	3	4	5

1. I really felt as if my physiotherapist/sport therapist understood the concerns I have about the injury.

    1   2   3   4   5

2. I felt free to talk to my physiotherapist/sport therapist about the things that were bothering me.

    1   2   3   4   5

3. The physiotherapist/sport therapist was very sensitive towards my needs as an active person.

    1   2   3   4   5

*4. I felt that this physiotherapist/sport therapist wasn't as sympathetic towards my injury as I would have liked.

    1   2   3   4   5

5. I felt that the physiotherapist/sport therapist tried to understand how the injury may affect my involvement in sport.

    1   2   3   4   5

6. The physiotherapist/sport therapist gave me a chance to say what was really on my mind.

    1   2   3   4   5

7. After talking with the physiotherapist/sport therapist I now know much more about the severity of my injury.

    1   2   3   4   5

8. After talking with the physiotherapist/sport therapist I have a better idea of how long the injury rehabilitation process should take.

    1   2   3   4   5

9. The physiotherapist/sport therapist told me all I wanted to know about my injury.

    1   2   3   4   5

*10. The physiotherapist/sport therapist explained the nature of my injury in words that were difficult to understand.

    1   2   3   4   5

11. The diagnosis of my injury was made following a thorough and careful examination.

    1   2   3   4   5

12. The physiotherapist/sport therapist appeared competent during the examination.

        1   2   3   4   5

13. The physiotherapist/sport therapist didn't seem at all rushed during the examination of my injury.

        1   2   3   4   5

*Item reverse-coded.

NB—Items:

1–6   perceived empathy shown by physiotherapist;

7–10   perceived quality of information given;

11–13   perceived competence of physiotherapist.

7 *Managing thoughts, stress, and pain*

Jane Crossman

In the sport psychology literature there is a well-known adage that states: 'how you think is how you perform'. For injured athletes, the phrase can be translated to 'how you think can affect how you progress in rehabilitation'. The thoughts that injured athletes have regarding their injury will influence their perception of it and its potential impact on their future athletic careers, their lives, and the length of time it takes to make a successful return to action. Negative mental preoccupations almost always affect stress levels and may lead to physical reactions such as muscle tension and pain.

Self-talk

Self-talk is an internal dialogue athletes are engaged in, which determines their interpretation of the situation and, in turn, their physical and psychological reaction to it. There are two types of self-talk: positive and negative. It is probable that in the early stages of rehabilitation athletes' internal dialogue may be largely composed of negative statements. Examples of negative self-statements follow:

'I'm never going to get back to where I was.'

'This rehab is useless. I'd be better off sitting at home watching television.'

'Being away from training sucks. Why did it have to happen to me?'

'I can't stand this pain anymore.'

As you can tell from the above examples, negative self-talk involves critical, self-demeaning, self-defeating, counterproductive thoughts, which will only serve to decrease effort in rehabilitation, decrease self-esteem, and increase anxiety, feelings of helplessness, and levels of depression.

Negative cognitions begin with a stressor (pain) and then the pain is influenced by the athletes' belief system ('I'm not going to be able to play/practice tomorrow.'). What then typically follows are negative feelings such as anger, frustration, and anxiety—often followed by a response such as catastrophizing ('The coach is going to dump me.') Clearly, the thought content of injured athletes influences recovery and therefore changing negative thinking into positive is important.

Positive self-talk or affirmations, which are really just mental pats on the back, serve to motivate the athlete to work through rehabilitation with confidence and sustained effort. Examples of positive self-statements follow:

'I'm getting stronger everyday.'

'I know I can get back to practice and competition if I work hard in rehab.'

'I have confidence that my sport therapist knows what she's doing.'

Encourage your clients to write down, on a card or in a logbook, a list of personal affirmations. These positive self-statements should be read several times each day or when they feel they need a reminder to think positively. Because positive thoughts are the kind that will assist athletes in making a successful recovery[1] and negative ones are counterproductive, it is important to educate athletes to replace negative, unproductive, intrusive thoughts with positive, productive ones. The idea here is that it is impossible to think of two contradictory thoughts at the same time.

The process of changing negative thoughts to positive is commonly called 'thought-stopping' and involves stopping a negative thought and replacing it with a positive one using a mental cue. It rose out of the need for more sophisticated ways of telling the athlete simply not to engage in negative thinking. Knowing that your clients are 'worrying about nothing', even knowing that their worries are false or unlikely to come true may not be sufficient to actually stop them.

Steps in thought-stopping

1. *Educational phase*: Talk to your athletes about the detrimental effects of negative thoughts and the importance of replacing negative thoughts with positive ones.

2. *Awareness phase*: Have athletes monitor and then write down the actual content of their negative thoughts on the left-hand side of a sheet of paper. Then on the right-hand side of the paper have them record a corresponding positive thought or what they would rather be saying to themselves. The positive thought should have the following features:
   - it should be opposite to or conflict with the negative thought;
   - it should be true, or at least more probable and realistic;
   - it should be assertive;
   - it should be positive.

   Examples are given in Table 7.1.

3. *Implementation phase*: First, athletes must recognize that they have had a negative thought. Once recognized, have them use a cue or trigger such

Table 7.1 Awareness phase

Negative thoughts	Positive thoughts
Rehab's such a waste of time.	At the end of every session I'm always glad I came.
I can't lift nearly as much as I used to.	I'm getting stronger all the time.
I'm totally useless.	I can at least help the team out by…
My knee's never going to heal.	My physician told me that my knee would heal but it would just take time and patience.

as a stop sign or the word 'stop' to halt the thought **each and every time** it occurs. Then change the negative thought to a positive one. The overriding principle is that injured athletes must never be allowed to finish the negative thought. Thought-stopping can be even more effective if combined with a physical reminder such as stomping the floor.

Other strategies to modify thought content

There are other techniques athletes can implement to get rid of unwanted negative thinking. Have them:

- imagine writing the negative thought on a piece of paper, crumpling it up, and throwing it in the garbage can;
- imagine writing the negative thought on a sheet of paper, putting it into an envelope, sealing it, and mailing it;
- image that the negative thought is contained inside a helium balloon, then ask them to let go of the balloon and watch as it sails into the air and far away;
- imagine putting each negative image into a file, then placing it in a filing cabinet closing the drawer.

Thinking rationally

Whenever athletes experience a negative emotional outcome in response to being injured, there is a tendency to attribute the cause of the reaction to whatever or whoever they feel was responsible. While these reactions (both emotional and rational) are often affected by prior learning and personal experience, it is important for athletes to realize that it is not external events which caused the reaction but rather their perceptions of it. The skill of rational thinking is based on Dr Albert Ellis' approach to problem-solving called rational-emotive therapy.[2]

Whenever athletes experience some stressor, such as being reprimanded by their physician for lifting too much weight too early in the rehabilitation process, they do not react immediately (although it may seem so) but rather actively interpret what is being said or done. In other words, they engage in self-talk. Following that, the body responds in some way (muscle tension), and then feelings may be aroused. Then, and only then, do athletes respond. It is possible that athletes may react to the same stressor differently when presented on two different occasions, depending on their psychological state. A major factor influencing their personal reactions to any situation is the role their beliefs (i.e., perceptions, opinions, attitudes) play. Beliefs about events are key factors influencing the content of self-talk. In some cases, however, beliefs about things are based on partial truths or falsehoods which go unchallenged and which may influence their reaction to their injury.

Some injured athletes may have a tendency to either exaggerate the extent of their injury (e.g., a wrestler turning a sprained elbow into a dislocated one) or downplay it (e.g., continuing to run even though experiencing persistent pain because of shin splints). Two of my early studies[3,4] found that athletes who are likely to exaggerate the seriousness of their injury tend to be more novice athletes performing at lower levels.

Athletes who think irrationally use words such as 'must' and 'have to'. They also tend to catastrophize and put themselves and others down. Typical irrational beliefs (sometimes called cognitive distortions) might be: 'I must get back to training'; 'My injury is unbearable'; 'It's my coach's fault that I'm injured'; 'I must be valued by all my teammates'. These sort of statements will only lead to exaggerated, non-productive results.

Medical practitioners can help athletes modify these faulty beliefs. First, these beliefs must be detected, and the best way to achieve that is by the process of self-monitoring. Have athletes document their self-talk as it occurs in reaction to stressful events. By doing this they will likely determine that their self-talk is closely linked with the feelings experienced. Then the irrational belief must be challenged. For example, ask them what evidence they have that: 'I'll never be able to row again'. After some internal debate they may come to realize that there is little evidence to support their contention.

Another way of challenging these irrational beliefs is to examine carefully the words that are being used. For example, a client may say, 'My coach *always* makes me feel useless'. The word 'always' is an absolute. Logically speaking, nothing 'always' happens. Suggest to athletes that they soften words such as 'have to', 'must', 'should', 'never' by replacing them with words and phrases such as 'would like to', 'it might be nice if' and 'sometimes'. In other words, their internal dialogue becomes more moderate and realistic. Hence, behavior becomes based on facts instead of feelings and becomes more productive.

In numerous discussions with injured athletes, I've noticed that some tend to overgeneralize their thoughts regarding their injury. 'Every time I mention my injury to my parents they tell me it's all in my head' is an example. Even if the event happened once or twice, the athlete may jump to the conclusion that this is a regular occurrence.

Likewise, some injured athletes see everything in terms of black and white, or all or nothing. For example, an athlete either loves or hates his therapist, or a coach is either good or bad. This stringent kind of thinking is illogical. Real life is filled with shades of grey.

Helping athletes think in clear, positive, and logical ways involves confronting their beliefs with real evidence. A basketball player with torn ankle ligaments may say to you: 'I've got to get back to practice or the coach will drop me from the team'. Ask her whether the coach actually said that this would happen. Likely not.

The bottom line is that external events and persons cannot make injured athletes think in ways that will impede recovery. They, and they alone, control how they think and what they believe to be true. With this understanding, medical practitioners can assist their clients by teaching them to think in positive, realistic, and constructive ways that direct them towards achieving their goals in rehabilitation.

Relaxation

Numerous sport psychologists and medical practitioners support the contention that participating in a systematic program of relaxation can be of tremendous value to injured athletes in the process of recovery.[5–8] Indeed, numerous high-performance athletes use a variety of forms of relaxation to help them achieve an 'Ideal performance state'. Relaxation typically lowers heart rate, breathing, metabolic rate, and blood pressure.[9] With regard to its role in rehabilitation, relaxation can reduce muscle tension which, in turn, reduces the amount of pain experienced.[10] Relaxation is a technique that reduces the feelings of frustration, depression, and anger which often accompany the onset of injury.[11]

The cornerstone of modern relaxation techniques is progressive relaxation, introduced by the physiologist Edmund Jacobson in 1938.[12] In recent years it has been modified to make it simpler and more effective. Relaxation is a temporary and deliberate withdrawal from everyday activity that moderates the sympathetic nervous system functions, which are usually activated by stressful situations, e.g. having to cope with negative emotional reactions as a result of being injured. Relaxation can also help athletes conserve vital energy required to promote healing and fight disease, control pain, and that may assist those who are having trouble sleeping. Progressive muscular relaxation (PMR) consists of learning to sequentially tense and then relax various groups of muscles all through the body, while at the same time paying very close and careful attention to the feelings associated with both tension and relaxation. Thus, PMR will help your client to learn to recognize and pin-point tension and relaxation as they appear in injury-specific situations as well as everyday situations. The goal of relaxation training is to help your clients learn to reduce muscle tension far below the adaptation level (day-to-day) at any time they wish.

Learning to relax

When learning to relax, athletes pass through three levels of relaxation. As they pass through these levels, their state of relaxation increases and their sense of control heightens. The levels are as follows:

1. *The symbolic level*—at this initial level, the athletes' breathing will slow down and deepen and they will begin to realize that they create tension or relaxation.

2. *The mental level*—a sense of calm begins to envelope them and because athletes now begin to focus their attention away from anxiety-causing distractions, they reassert control over themselves.

3. *The physical level*—athletes become able to evoke a deep relaxed state through practice, which allows them to have control over any cognitive (mental) or somatic (physical) anxieties which may be impeding recovery.

Procedures

The environment in which the relaxation takes place is an important consideration. For that reason, a quiet, comfortable atmosphere with subdued lighting should be provided. The athletes should be positioned comfortably in a chair or lying down, with clothes loosened and shoes off. Ask them to close their eyes and take several deep abdominal breaths. Instruct them to concentrate on how their body feels and rid the mind of all other thoughts. At this point, they may be asked to scan the body for tension, to determine which areas are particularly tight or tense.

In PMR, muscle groups are tensed and relaxed in a systematic fashion. Tensing muscles prior to letting them relax is like giving the muscles a running start toward relaxation through the momentum created by the tension release (similar to drawing back a pendulum before letting it go). The tension phase will also allow the athlete the opportunity to feel the distinction between the feeling of tension and relaxation because the two responses are mutually exclusive (i.e., it is not possible to be relaxed and tense at the same time).

Guidelines when implementing PMR

- *Breathing*—after the first initial deep breaths, subsequent breaths should be steady and shallow. Inhalations and exhalations should be through the nose.

- *Tension phase*—this should last approximately 7–10 seconds. With a slightly raised voice, include phrases such as: 'hold the tension in the muscles', 'feel the tension and hold it', 'you may notice some feelings of tightness or strain in these muscles'.

- *Relaxation phase*—should last approximately 25–30 seconds. With a lowered tone of voice (compared to the tension phase), include words and phrases such as: 'calm' and 'relaxed', 'concentrate on the difference between the feel of tension and relaxation', 'feel the relief of letting go', 'feel the heaviness and warmth in the muscles', 'no effort, no tension', 'concentrate on the feeling of letting go'.

As previously indicated, muscles are tensed and relaxed in a systematic fashion. I start with the arms, then move to the head, neck and shoulders, abdomen then legs. I recommend that 16 muscle groups be initially relaxed and when your athlete can relax them without difficulty then the length of each session can be cut down by combining groups of muscles to seven then four. The sequencing of muscle groups and corresponding actions to contract muscles are as follows:

16 muscle groups:
1. Right hand and forearm—make a tight fist with the right hand.
2. Right upper arm and bicep region—push the right arm into the side of the body and into the back of a chair (or floor).
3. Left hand and forearm—make a tight fist with the left hand.
4. Left upper arm—push the left arm into the side of the body and into the back of the chair.
5. Forehead area—raise the eyebrows, make a deep frown.
6. Eyes and nose—squint hard and wrinkle the nose.
7. Mouth and jaw area—clench the teeth hard and force the lips back.
8. Neck—push the head back into the chair and raise the shoulders up.
9. Shoulders and chest—take a deep breath and draw the shoulder blades back and together.
10. Abdomen—tighten the muscles by sucking in.
11. Upper right leg—raise the right leg off the chair (or floor) about 10 centimeters (4 inches).
12. Right calf—point the right toes up (dorsi flex).
13. Right foot and toes—curl the right toes and point the foot inward.
14. Upper left thigh—raise the right leg off the chair about 10 centimeters.
15. Left calf—point the left toes (dorsi flex).
16. Left foot and toes—curl the left toes and point the foot inward.

7 muscle groups

1. Right arm—make a tight fist and push the right arm into the side and back of the chair.
2. Left arm—make a tight fist and push the left arm into the side and back of the chair.
3. Face—raise the eyebrows and draw the lips back.
4. Neck and shoulders—raise the shoulders and draw the shoulder blades back and together.
5. Torso—tighten the chest and abdominal muscles by sucking in.
6. Right leg and foot—raise the leg about 10 centimeters off the chair and point the toes.
7. Left leg and feet—raise the leg about 10 centimeters off the chair and point the toes.

4 muscle groups

1. Both hands and arms—clench both fists and draw the arms into the side and back of the chair.
2. Face, neck, and shoulders—raise the eyebrows, draw the lips back, lift the shoulders and push them into the back of the chair.
3. Torso—tighten the chest and abdominal muscles by sucking in.
4. Feet and legs—raise both legs about 10 centimeters and point the toes.

    *   *Cue words and phrases*—when athletes are in a relaxed state (i.e., after 16, 7, or 4 muscle groups), I incorporate at this time a cue word (usually 'calm') and say it repeatedly with every exhalation for about 1 minute. Then I instruct them to continue saying the word 'calm' to themselves so that they begin to associate the word 'calm' with the feeling of relaxation. Practiced often enough, through the process of classical conditioning, the athlete will be able to relax quickly by saying the word 'calm' (in conjunction with some deep inhalations) to ward off unwanted anxiety before, for example, a doctor's appointment, going to rehabilitation, or even prior to surgery.
    *   *Ending the session*—to end each session I tell the athletes that I will count backwards from 3 to 1 and when I say: 'three', move their legs; 'two', move their arms; and 'one', open their eyes. This technique avoids ending the session abruptly and hopefully leaves them feeling refreshed and relaxed.

Scanning

Scanning involves having athletes note signs of muscular tension during the day. For example, teeth may be clenched or neck and shoulder muscles tight.

By scanning the body at least twice a day, they will then be able to implement the relaxation response in a short time by deep breathing or autogenic training.

Autogenic training

Another technique that injured athletes may find effective for eliciting a relaxed state of being, thereby promoting healing is autogenic training (AT) meaning 'self-generated'.[13] What differentiates this technique from others, including PMR, is that it utilizes self-hypnosis and doesn't require any physical activity, which would likely be preferred for those athletes who are in pain or immobile.

Autogenic training emphasizes two bodily sensations: heaviness in the limbs; and warmth in the body, arms, and legs. Body warmth is caused by blood vessels dilating, resulting in an increase in blood flow. Heaviness in the limbs is caused by muscles relaxing in association with verbal cues such as 'heavy', 'warm', and 'relaxed'.

While AT has many physiological benefits (including decreased heart rate, respiratory rate, muscle tension, serum cholesterol level), there are numerous psychological benefits as well (including increased pain tolerance, resistance to stress and decreased depression, fear and anxiety).

Athletes should be comfortable, either sitting on a bench (arms resting on thighs), in an easy chair, or reclined (lying on back). Instruct them to begin by taking some deep diaphragmatic breaths. To accomplish this have them imagine the lungs are divided into three sections: the lower, middle, and upper. Have them try and fill the lower section first by pushing the diaphragm down and forcing the abdomen out. The middle section can be then filled with air by expanding the chest cavity and raising the ribcage. Finally, the upper section of the lungs is filled by raising the shoulders and chest.

AT is a six-stage process. Athletes shouldn't move to the next stage until the previous one is well learned. The stages and sample autosuggestions are as follows:

1. Heaviness in the arms and legs, beginning with the dominant arm or leg. 'My right leg is very heavy.'
2. Warmth in the arms and legs, beginning with the dominant arm or leg. 'My left arm feels very warm.'
3. Warmth in the chest to regulate the heart rate. 'The muscles in my chest are warm and my heart is beating quietly.'
4. Regulation of breathing. 'My breathing rate is regular, slow, and relaxed.'
5. Warmth in the solar plexus. With hand on the upper abdominal area say, 'My solar plexus feels warm.'

6. Coolness in the forehead. 'My forehead feels cool.'

The next stage is to combine AT with imagery (see below). For example, athletes could help facilitate healing or increase pain tolerance by combining images of seeing the body repairing (mending broken bones) with feelings of heaviness and warmth in the arms and legs. Finally, they can utilize self-statements to suggest to the mind that the body is healing and better prepared to handle pain.

One final note

With PMR and AT it's important that you tell your clients not to expect instant results. Only with practice will total relaxation be achieved. There are numerous guided relaxation and autogenic training audiotapes available. If you wish, you may make your own tape for your clients.

In the early stages of learning PMR a full session should be undertaken every day for several weeks. Then as clients become more familiar and comfortable with the procedure, they may begin to stretch the schedule. AT requires approximately 15 minutes per session and ideally is performed twice a day for several months. This relaxation technique may therefore be unsuitable for athletes wanting quicker results. Once mastered, your clients will be able to elicit the relaxation response in minutes.

Imagery

Imagery (also referred to as visualization or mental practice/rehearsal) involves using all the senses (seeing, hearing, smelling, tasting, and feeling) to create or re-create an experience in the mind.[14] Well-supported results show that while injured athletes may be unable to physically practice, they can instead harness the power of their own private imagination

Imagery has been the subject of numerous studies for over 80 years, and meta-analyses have been conducted regarding its application.[15] Many sport psychologists and medical practitioners have documented their belief in the potential value of imagery[6,16–20] and its ability to speed up the recovery process,[1,18,21,22] and even be used as a tool for prevention.[23] In many instances, practitioners have successfully combined a program of relaxation with imagery to enhance recovery following surgery.[17] Research has demonstrated that greater blood flow and warmth to the injured area (thereby promoting healing) has been facilitated by imagery.[24] It should be stated, however, that testimonies supporting the use of imagery as a tool to enhance and even speed up healing are anecdotal in nature and no direct link has been empirically established.

Neuromuscular and cognitive theories have been developed to explain why imagery works, including: the psychoneuromuscular theory;[25,26] the symbolic learning theory;[27] attentional–arousal set;[28] and the bioinformational theory.[29,30] It is beyond the scope of this chapter to overview each theory. In brief, imaging is akin to athletes having a virtual reality system in their heads. Further reading is encouraged for readers wishing to understand each theory (see the Further reading list at the end of this chapter).

Uses of imagery for injured athletes

Injured athletes can make different mental images, with the purposes of helping them:

- heal, e.g. broken bones, torn ligaments;[1,21,31]
- make mental pictures of themselves getting better or recovering, i.e. stronger, more flexible;[18]
- replace the physical practice lost during rehabilitation;[32]
- mentally practice skills and strategies they have learned prior to becoming injured;
- improve confidence and remain positive about their recovery;
- control negative emotional disturbance and anxiety which often accompany injury;
- control pain[33] and cope with it.[34,35]

Guidelines

1. Injured athletes should visualize at least once a day for 15 minutes during the time they are rehabilitating from their injury. When beginning a program of relaxation, athletes should keep their images short in duration but frequent, i.e., daily.

2. Imaging should be done in a quiet, comfortable environment. Before beginning, have clients take a few slow, controlled, deep breaths to clear the mind and relax.

3. Clients can opt to visualize externally (as if on video) or internally (as if they were actually physically doing the activity or looking from inside to the outside world). Research shows that higher level performers tend to visualize more internally,[1,36] although many can readily switch back and forth from internal to external.

4. Injured athletes should always visualize positive or successful performances. For example, the weight should be lifted, the stretch done correctly, or the pass made.

5. In the early stages of learning, it may be necessary to have the client verbalize each scene before concentrating on it. The verbalization may be a good strategy to foster communication between the athlete and medical professional treating the injury.

6. Have athletes stimulate as many senses as possible, including visual, olfactory, auditory, tactile, gustatory, and kinesthetic; by doing this they can create and re-create the environment as vividly as possible. In other words, have them see the ski moguls, smell the chlorine, hear the sound of the ball leaving the bat, feel the water, and taste the salty sweat, etc.

7. Encourage athletes to focus on the 'feel' of the movements. They may wish to sit up or re-create the motions they actually perform when physically practicing.[37]

8. Don't allow athletes to speed up their images. Most athletes see their images in real time but some prefer to visualize as if the action was being performed in slow motion.

9. Avoid images that anticipate reinjury or negatively recall the occurrence of the present injury because they can have an adverse effect on recovery rate.[38]

   The following are examples of some healing images your athletes can use:

   • blood flowing to the muscle, rebuilding it at an accelerated rate during resistance training;

   • ice as freezing up and shutting down pain receptors;

   • deep breathing to infuse the body with healing energy.

An imagery program

A four-step process of imagery implementation has been developed by Richardson and Latuda.[1] The steps include:

1. *Introducing imagery*—This involves defining what imagery is and a brief explanation of how it's done. Because it is important for the athlete to believe that imagery can really help in the rehabilitative process, it would be prudent to point out that research shows the vast majority of high-performance athletes visualize.[39]

2. *Evaluating the athlete's ability to visualize*—At this point it's important to determine your client's ability to visualize. For example, have the athlete imagine an orange or a campfire and to bring into that image as many senses as possible. It's a good idea to remind the athlete that images can be both internal and external and that some athletes can even alternate between both.

3. *Developing basic imagery*—Have athletes practice twice a day for 15 minutes, dividing each session into three phases: (1) vividness, (2) controllability, and (3) self-perception.

It is recommended that the vividness phase occurs for at least 5 minutes. This phase involves picking a basic skill and going over it in the mind, feeling the muscles work and the sensations that normally occur when the skill is performed. Then as they master visualizing basic skills, more complex ones can be added to their imagery repertoire.

Controllability involves visualizing a basic skill, but this time in conjunction with teammates or the opposition. By doing this, strategies and plays can be mentally rehearsed even though the injured athlete is unable to physically practice them with the team. To be able to learn new team strategies, it is recommended that injured athletes attend as many practices and team meetings as possible. By doing so, feelings of being ostracized from the team may also be reduced. Also, it is hoped that ongoing performance-related images will pave the way for a smooth and confident transition back into practice and competition.

In the self-perception phase, have athletes visualize a superior performance from their past athletic careers—perhaps a personal best or a performance far above expectation. Then ask them to isolate the characteristics which made that performance superior, considering the precompetition and competition thoughts and actions.

4. *Using imagery in rehabilitative programs*— During this final phase you should explain to your clients what their injury is in terms they can understand. Augmenting your explanation with pictures, radiographs, etc. would be useful. Then have them make a vivid mental picture of the injury, followed by having them make a mental image of that injury being repaired. For example, torn ligaments growing on to the bone or sponges acting as anti-inflammatory medication. As time passes and recovery progresses, athletes should make images that reflect healing.

Systematic desensitization

I've counselled athletes who have a fear of returning to practice and competition for fear of reinjury. They remember vividly what happened and how they felt at the time of the onset of their injury (in the case of an acute injury), and invariably they remember the pain associated with the trauma. This association between the activity (e.g., falling while skiing down an icy slope, crashing into a goalpost (before the advent of mag-nets)) and the pain experienced was indelible; so much so that it was preventing them from returning to their sports.

One technique I've found effective for helping athletes overcome such fears is systematic desensitization (SD). SD, developed by Wolpe[40] was originally a clinical procedure for the treatment of phobias such as flying in airplanes or public speaking. By pairing relaxation or a state of calmness with images of the anxiety-provoking behavior (skating towards a goalpost, skiing down an icy slope), the connection between the stimulus and response will be weakened. This deconditioning of the anxiety is commonly referred to as counter-conditioning and its usefulness has been supported in a case study.[41]

Steps

1. Athletes must recognize that they have a fear which is preventing them from fully participating in the sport.

2. Ask them to describe a number of situations that are related to the anxiety-provoking situation and rate each situation on a scale from 0 (comfortable/relaxed) to 10 (extremely tense/anxious). Then rank these situations by intensity of anxiousness (least to most) to create an anxiety or fear hierarchy.

3. Start by having them visualize, as vividly as possible, the least anxiety-provoking situation. Pair the visual image with a relaxation procedure. When they can imagine the situation and remain in a relaxed state (which is incompatible with fear), then, and only then, should you have them image the next situation in the hierarchy. Have them then work up the hierarchy (pairing imagery and relaxation) in a step-by-step fashion until they are able to overcome feelings of anxiety when presented with the situation that has been identified as the root of their fear. This may take numerous sessions.

Ideally the sessions are led by a person trained to provide both verbal instruction (i.e. when and what to visualize) and relaxation. The ultimate scenario occurs when they are able to actually go and do (not just visualize) the feared activity. Initially, the person who has been leading the systematic desensitization sessions should be present in case the athlete has difficulty transferring what has been visualized in a relaxed state to real life.

Non-pharmacological ways of managing pain

Managing pain is one of the challenges presented to injured athletes and those recovering from surgery. Following injury, athletes differ in their ability to cope with pain. The inability to control pain can have negative repercussions on recovery and returning to sport, and is associated with sport rehabilitation adherence.[42] From an informational perspective, pain may be beneficial when it alerts athletes to overtraining or damage that has already occurred.[33]

The International Association for the Study of Pain[43] refers to pain as both a 'sensory and emotional experience', which implies that pain has both psychological and physical properties. It is then logical that the effective treatment of pain can not only encompass both the traditional pharmacological methods but non-pharmacological ones as well. Non-pharmacological techniques that have proven successful in the control of pain and which medical practitioners can teach their clients include: deep breathing, relaxation, imagery, self-talk, and stress inoculation training (SIT). One study found that a 9-week, cognitive–behavioral treatment program consisting of relaxation training, goal-setting, medication reduction, coping skills training, activity pacing, and anxiety and mood management was effective in reducing chronic pain.[44] Some pain management strategies are best implemented by those with specialized training. For example, a sport psychologist or registered psychologist should be recruited to conduct sessions in hypnosis, meditation, transcendental meditation, biofeedback; and a registered massage therapist to deliver massage therapy.

Melzack and Wall[45] through their Gate Control Theory were the first to acknowledge that pain had a psychological component. The Parallel Processing Model[46] posits that pain is impacted by two psychological influences: information and emotion. Their empirical investigations found that people experience significantly less pain when they attend to the informational aspects of it (cause, location, and sensory characteristics) than when they pay attention to the emotional characteristics (fear, avoidance, or distress).

There are two types of pain: acute and chronic. Acute is intense and short in duration and is likely the result of a sudden traumatic event, such as getting a 'stitch' in the side while running. Chronic pain is constant and persists for a long time after the onset of injury. It's important for athletes to learn to read the signals that the pain is sending. For example, pain experienced while lifting weights during physical therapy may be a signal to cut back until more healing has occurred. To reduce anxiety associated with the injury *per se* and the subsequent pain that may be experienced, it is advised that the medical practitioner inform athletes about what is causing pain, what sensations may be experienced as an outcome of the injury or surgery, and, finally, strategies for pain reduction. Depending on the medical practitioner's level of understanding and available time he/she may wish to take on the responsibility of educating the athlete and conducting the sessions or to refer the athlete to a sport psychologist.

Non-pharmacological, pain management strategies have been classified into two categories: pain reduction and pain focusing.[16] Pain reduction techniques reduce the sympathetic nervous system responses that increase pain, these methods include deep breathing, PMR, meditation, and therapeutic massage. Pain focusing techniques direct attention into (associative) and away from (dissociative) the pain to decrease it.

Pain reduction strategies

Abdominal breathing
This simple, yet effective, technique is easily learned by athletes to reduce tension and manage pain and is particularly effective during acute pain flares.

To heal efficiently, athletes need a greater than usual amount of oxygen. Abdominal breathing involves a long, slow inhalation that fills the chest, holding that inhalation for a few seconds, and then slowly exhaling.

To facilitate greater breathing awareness, have athletes perform the following steps:

1. Lie down on a cushioned floor or table with legs and arms uncrossed and eyes closed.

2. Scan the body for tension.

3. Bring attention to breathing by placing the hand on the abdomen (if the upper chest is rising and falling it is likely that the breaths are quick and shallow and consequently not reflective of deep abdominal breathing).

4. Breathe through the nose.

5. Use imagery to facilitate deep abdominal breathing.

Turk, Meichenbaum, and Genest[47] described the following image to facilitate slow inhalations and exhalations: 'As you exhale slowly, imagine that you are gently blowing across the top of a spoon of hot soup so you do not spill it or that you are flickering a candle without blowing it out'.

Have athletes monitor their pain and tension levels several times a day. Because abdominal breathing can be done virtually anywhere at almost anytime, it serves as an effective means of managing pain and reducing tension.

Stress inoculation training

Stress Inoculation Training (SIT) is a cognitive–behavioral intervention program that links relaxation, self-talk, and attention-diversion, including imagery.[48] SIT can be of value to injured athletes as a means of managing pain.[49,50] SIT is composed of three phases: conceptualization, skill acquisition, and rehearsal. In the conceptualization phase the injured athlete gains a greater understanding of the effects of stress (pain) upon emotions and performance. Next is the skill acquisition phase where athletes learn to self-monitor cognitive and emotional indicators of pain using physical-based coping skills. At this time athletes are allowed to choose the coping techniques they wish to employ, such as relaxation, deep breathing, distraction, imagery, and positive self-statements. In the final phase, athletes rehearse these pain management strategies several times a day and specifically when they are experiencing pain.

Pain focusing techniques

Pain focusing has been divided into two categories: associative and dissociative.[51] Associative focusing involves attending to particular aspects of pain. This can involve either focusing on bodily sensations to localize the pain and restrict its usual global nature, or reappraising the pain into positive terms. By having athletes monitor their internal states, they may be able to control the intensity, location, and meaning of the pain. Dissociation involves focusing away from the pain and involves either internal distractors (imagining a pleasant walk, counting, or repeating a word or phrase) or external distractors (watching television or a video, or listening to music).

Research has shown that the use of dissociative strategies is better for acute pain and minor injuries involving a short period of rehabilitation, i.e. a week or two.

Association may be more appropriate for chronic pain and injuries requiring lengthy rehabilitation, i.e., more than 2 weeks.[52]

When rehabilitation necessitates concentrating on the task at hand, as in strength training, then diverting attention away (dissociating) may be dangerous because athletes might not pick up pain messages (such as ease up or slow down), which could result in further injury.

Acknowledgements

The author would like to thank Trish McGowan, Amy M. Gayman, Sarah Gee and Paulene T. McGowan for their critiques of the preliminary drafts of this chapter.

Further reading

Achterberg, J., Dossey, B., and Kolkneier, L. (1994). *Rituals of healing: Using imagery for health and wellness.* Bantam Books, New York.

Benson, H. and Stuart, E. (1992). *The wellness book: The comprehensive guide to maintaining health and treating stress-related illness.* Birch Lane, Secaucus, NJ.

Coleman, D. and Green, J. (ed.) (1993). *Mind body medicine: How to use your mind for better health.* Consumer Report Books, Yonkers, NY.

Cox, R. H. (1998). *Sport psychology: Concepts and applications*, pp. 172–80. MCB McGraw-Hill, Boston, MA.

Davis, M., Eschelman, E., and McKay, M. (1995). *The relaxation and stress reduction workbook* (4th edn). New Harbinger, Oakland, CA.

References

1. Richardson, P. A. and Latuda, L. M. (1995). Therapeutic imagery and athletic injuries. *Journal of Athletic Training*, **30**, 10–12.
2. Ellis, A. (1970). *The essence of rational psychotherapy: a comprehensive approach to treatment.* Institute for Rational Living, New York.

3. Crossman, J. and Jamieson, J. (1985). Differences in perceptions of seriousness and disrupting effects of athletic injury as viewed by athletes and their trainer. *Perceptual and Motor Skills*, **61**, 1131–4.

4. Crossman, J., Jamieson, J., and Hume, K. M. (1990). Perceptions of athletic injuries by athletes, coaches, and medical professionals, *Perceptual and Motor Skills*, **71**, 848–50.

5. Gieck, J. (1990). Psychological consideration of rehabilitation. In *Rehabilitation techniques in sports medicine* (ed. W. Prentice), pp. 107–122. Times Mirror/Mosby, Toronto.

6. Pargman, D. (ed.) (1993). *Psychological bases of sport injuries*. Fitness Information Technology, Morgantown, West Virginia.

7. Carroll, S. A. (1993). Mental imagery as an aid to healing the injured athlete. Unpublished master's thesis, San Diego State University, CA.

8. Davis, M. E., Eschelman, E., and McKay, M. (1995). *The relaxation and stress reduction workbook* (4th edn). New Harbinger, Oakland, CA.

9. Benson, H., Beary, J. F., and Carol, M. D. (1974). The relaxation response. *Psychiatry*, **37**, 37–46.

10. Linton, S. J. and Gotestam, K. G. (1984). A controlled study of the effects of applied relaxation and applied relaxation plus operant procedures in regulation of chronic pain. *British Journal of Clinical Psychology*, **23**, 291–9.

11. Crossman, J. (1997) Psychological rehabilitation from sports injuries. *Sports Medicine*, **23**, 333–9.

12. Jacobson, E. (1938). *Progressive relaxation* (2nd edn). University of Chicago Press, Chicago.

13. Schultz, J. H. and Luthe, W. (1959). *Autogenic training*. Grune and Stratton, New York.

14. Veally, R. S. and Greenleaf, C. S. (1998). Seeing is believing: Understand and using imagery in sport. In *Applied sport psychology* (3rd edn) (ed. J. Williams), p. 238. Mayfield Publishing, Co., CA.

15. Feltz, D. L. and Landers, D. M. (1983). The effects of mental practice on motor skill learning and performance: A meta-analysis. *Journal of Sport Psychology*, **5**, 25–57.

16. Heil, J. (ed.) (1993). *Psychology of sport injury*. Human Kinetics, Champaign, IL.

17. Durso-Cupal, D. D. (1996). The efficacy of guided imagery for recovery from anterior cruciate ligament (ACL) replacement. *Journal of Applied Sport Psychology*, **8**(Suppl.), S56.

18. Green, L. B. (1992). The use of imagery in the rehabilitation of injured athletes. *The Sport Psychologist*, **6**, 416–28.

19. Jones, L. and Stuth, G. (1997). The uses of mental imagery in athletics: An overview. *Applied and Preventive Psychology*, **6**, 101–15.

20. Brewer, B. W., Jeffers, K. E., Petitpas, A. J., and Van Raalte, J. L. (1994). Perceptions of psychological interventions in the context of sport injury rehabilitation. *The Sport Psychologist*, **8**, 176–88.

21. Ievleva, L. and Orlick. T. (1991). Mental links to enhanced healing: An exploratory study. *The Sport Psychologist*, **5**, 25–40.
22. Loundagin, C. and Fisher, L. (October, 1993). The relationship between mental skills and enhance injury rehabilitation. Paper presented at the *Annual Meeting of the Association for the Advancement of Applied Sport Psychology*, Montreal, Canada.
23. Davis, J. O. (1991). Sport injuries and stress management: An opportunity for research. *The Sport Psychologist*, **5**, 175–82.
24. Blakeslee, T. R. (1980). *The right brain*. Anchor Press, New York.
25. Jacobson, E. (1931). Electrical measurements of neuromuscular states during mental activities. *American Journal of Physiology*, **96**, 115–21.
26. Suinn, R. M. (1980). Psychology and sport performance: Principles and applications. In *Psychology in sports: methods and applications* (ed. R. M. Suinn), pp. 26–36. Burgess, Minneapolis, MN.
27. Sackett, R. S. (1935). The relationship between the amount of symbolic rehearsal and retention of a maze habit. *Journal of General Psychology*, **13**, 113–28.
28. Schmidt, R. A. (1982). *Motor control and learning: a behavioral emphasis.* Human Kinetics, Champaign, IL.
29. Lang, P. J. (1977). Imagery in therapy: An information processing analysis of fear. *Behavior Therapy*, **8**, 862–86.
30. Lang, P. J. (1979). A bio-infomational theory of emotional imagery. *Psychophysiology*, **16**, 495–512.
31. Surgent, F. S. (1991). Using your mind to beat injuries. *Running and FitNews*, **1**, 4–5.
32. Romero, K. and Silvestri, L. (1990). The role of mental practice in the acquisition and performance of motor skills. *Journal of Instructional Psychology*, **17**, 218–21.
33. Gauron, E. F. and Bowers, W. A. (1986). Pain control techniques in college-age athletes. *Psychological Reports*, **59**, 1163–9.
34. Achterberg, J., Kenner, C., and Lawlis, G. F. (1988). Severe burn injury: A comparison of relaxation, imagery, and biofeedback for pain management. *Journal of Mental Imagery*, **12**, 71–88.
35. Spanos, N. P. and O'Hara, P. A. (1990). Imaginal dispositions and situation-specific expectations in strategy-induced pain reductions. *Imagination, Cognition and Personality*, **9**, 147–56.
36. Mahoney, M. and Avener, M. (1977). Psychology of the elite athlete: An exploratory study. *Cognitive Therapy and Research*, **1**, 135–41.
37. Barr, K. and Hall, C. (1992). The use of imagery by rowers. *International Journal of Sport Psychology*, **23**, 242–61.
38. Grunert, B. K., Devine, C. A. Matloub, H. S. Sanger, J. R., and Yousif, N. J. (1988). Flashbacks after traumatic hand injuries: Prognostic indicators. *Journal of Hand Surgery*, **13**, 125–7.

39. Orlick, T. and Partington, J. (1988). Mental links to excellence. *The Sport Psychologist*, **2**, 105–30.

40. Wolpe, J. (1958). *Psychotherapy by reciprocal inhibition*. Stanford University Press, Stanford, CA.

41. Rotella, R. J. and Campbell, M. S. (1983). Systematic desensitization: Psychological rehabilitation of injured athletes. *Athletic Training*, **18**, 149–52.

42. Byerly, P. N., Worrell, T., Gahimer, J., and Domholdt, E. (1994). Rehabilitation compliance in an athletic training environment. *Journal of Athletic Training*, **29**, 352–5.

43. Merskey, H. and Bogduk, N. (eds). (1994). *Classification of chronic pain: Descriptions of chronic pain syndromes and definitions of pain terms* (2nd ed.) Seattle, WA: International Association for the Study of Pain Press.

44. Phillips, H. C. (1987). The effect of behavioural treatment on chronic pain. *Behavioural Research and Therapy*, **25**, 365–77.

45. Melzack, R. and Wall, P. D. (1965) Pain mechanisms: A new theory. *Science*, **150**, 971–9.

46. Leventhal, H. and Everhart, D. (1979) Emotion, pain, and physical illness. In *Emotions in personality and psychopathology* (ed. C. E. Izard), pp. 263–98. Plenum, New York.

47. Turk, D., Meichenbaum, D., and Genest, M. (1983). *Pain and behavioural medicine. A cognitive-behavioural perspective*. Guilford Press, New York.

48. Meichenbaum, D. (1985). *Stress inoculation training* Pergamon Press, New York.

49. Ross, M. J. and Berger, R. S. (1996). Effects of stress inoculation training on athletes' postsurgical pain and rehabilitation after orthopaedic injury. *Journal of Consulting and Clinical Psychology*, **64**, 406–10.

50. Whitmarsh, B. G. and Alderman, R. B. (1993). Role of psychological skills training in increasing athletic pain tolerance. *The Sport Psychologist*, **7**, 388–99.

51. Morgan, W. P. and Pollack, M. L. (1977). Psychological characterization of the elite distance runner. *Annals of the New York Academy of Science*, **301**, 382–403.

52. Suls, J. and Fletcher, B. (1985). The relative efficacy of avoidant and nonavoidant coping strategies: a meta-analysis. *Health Psychology*, **4**, 249–88.

8 The role of significant others: social support during injuries

Eileen Udry

Introduction

Consider the following quotes from a qualitative study of elite, injured ski athletes:[1]

> They [my parents] were totally supportive, but not able to be there physically [after my injury].
>
> Certain teammates were there through the injury ... they would fax me from wherever they were and let me know what the team was doing. That was really cool. But, definitely only some teammates—it's just the people that are closest to you.
>
> I think a big mistake that the coaching staff made when I was coming back [from my injury] was that they were always complimenting me. They were always telling me how well I was doing—which really boosted my ego—but it also added to the inability to cope with the obstacle [injury setback] that came up later. Their intentions were probably good, but I think, as a result, it affected the way I had to deal with my setbacks later on.
>
> He [my orthopedic surgeon] places so much trust in what you say. I mean he will ask you how it feels. I remember when it was my second time [injury]...I went in and he looked at me and said, 'When you fell, did it feel like a really bad injury?' And I said, 'Yeah.' And he said, 'Well, then it probably is.' So he placed his trust in me.

What do all of the above quotes have in common? Each illustrates that, while sport injuries happen to individual athletes, athletes' overall injury experience is significantly influenced—for better or worse—by those individuals who comprise athletes' social networks. Additionally, these quotes highlight some of the complexities of social support, and indicate that providing social support is more involved than merely 'complimenting' athletes on their rehabilitation progress. Clearly, there is a need for medical professionals and 'significant others' (referring here and throughout this chapter as family members, coaches, teammates) in injured athletes' social networks to understand how to provide social support, and for members of the network to effectively communicate this support. Thus, the overall purpose of this chapter is to discuss social support and its communication as it pertains to injured athletes' social networks. The chapter is divided into four sections. The first section defines and provides a conceptual overview of social support. The second section examines the role of three support providers—family members, coaches, and teammates—each of whom stands to play a potentially important role in the lives of injured athletes. The third section examines the effects of significant others on postinjury status (e.g., mental health functioning and adherence). The final section provides practical strategies for working and communicating with injured athletes' significant others.

Defining and conceptualizing social support: an optimal matching perspective

In the last several decades the way that social support is viewed has changed dramatically. Historically, Durkheim[2] is most often credited with providing the first empirical documentation of the influence of social support. Durkheim's work examined individuals' social ties in relation to suicide rates and found that suicide rates were higher among individuals who had few social ties. Durkheim concluded that a lack of social ties or *anomie* was contrary to psychological well-being. Although Durkheim's work stimulated a great deal of scientific exploration, social support is typically no longer viewed as simply the number of friendships or organizational ties.[3] Rather, what makes social support 'supportive' appears to be more related to the functional characteristics of an individual's social relationships (e.g., the quality or type of social support).[4] Thus, for example, in the case of injured athletes it's not how many teammates, family members, and friends stop by the hospital room after surgery that defines the injured athletes' social support levels. Rather, a better reflection would be what is communicated during the interactions injured athletes have with significant others during these hospital visits.

Since Durkheim's initial work, social support is a topic that has been widely researched and discussed.[2] There is, however, still no universally agreed upon definition of social support. One commonly accepted definition of social support is that it is an exchange of resources intended to benefit the recipient.[5] Thus, social support is viewed from the perspective of the support recipient. There is strong evidence for the idea that for the athlete to benefit from the support, the type, amount, and frequency of support must be matched to the needs or expectations of the athlete.[6–8] In other words, the right type of support must be provided, at the right time, and in the right amount—a phenomenon termed the 'optimal matching framework'.[6] Due to the practical relevance of the optimal matching framework relative to understanding social support and possible incongruencies in the provision and perceived usefulness of social support, the basic tenets of this framework will be described in more detail.

The right type of support

It has been repeatedly demonstrated that social support is a multidimensional construct and no type of support is universally preferred.[8-10] Thus, what is viewed as 'supportive' depends on a variety of factors including, but not limited to, the nature of the stressor and the individual. For instance, individuals experiencing a variety of health problems, such as cancer and migraine headaches, have been interviewed regarding the type of support they found helpful during their health difficulties. Patients experiencing these health difficulties have indicated three forms of social support are salient. These forms of social support include: esteem/emotional; informational; and tangible support. Esteem/emotional support included expressions of concern, empathy, and behaviors such as listening, physical presence, etc. Informational support was defined as information provided in an attempt to help individuals engage in problem-solving efforts, and included the provision of sound technical information. Tangible support encompassed effective practical assistance and the provision of technically competent medical care.

More recently, research has been conducted with injured athletes on the types of social support they found relevant during their injuries.[11] Interviews were conducted with over 50 athletes who had experienced relatively severe knee (i.e. anterior cruciate ligament) injuries. Athletes' responses supported the forms of social support noted above (i.e. esteem/emotional, informational, tangible), although a fourth type of social support also emerged as being relevant. This fourth type of support was termed 'motivational support', and referred to encouragement to overcome or acquiesce to obstacles or barriers. Motivational support was considered to be a significant form of support for athletes it as represented 24% of their reported social interactions. The fact there are differences across studies (i.e., patients with various health difficulties versus injured athletes) pertaining to the type of relevant support is viewed as evidence that there is no universally preferred type of social support. That is, the context of the situation and nature of the stressor should be taken into account when considering the relevant forms of social support.

Given the above information, from a practical perspective it is recommended that support providers attempt to match the type of support being provided with needs and preferences of the support recipient. (Further elaboration of the various forms of social support is provided in Table 8.1.) For instance, consider the example of an injured athlete who is seeking esteem/emotional support (e.g., an athlete wants her coach to appreciate how devastated she is over an injury). If the coach responds to the athlete with only informational support (i.e. 'most athletes are back from this injury in 6

Table 8.1 Components and examples of social support

Esteem/emotional	Reassuring behaviors communicating love and acceptance (e.g. physical presence, expressions of concern, empathy, affection, niceness, special understanding from others in similar circumstances)
Tangible	Provision of concrete assistance or goods (e.g. providing transportation to rehabilitation, fixing meals, assistance with financial or material concerns)
Informational	Information or advice targeted at problem-solving or feedback (e.g. providing advice, useful information, being a positive role model)
Motivational	Providing encouragement to overcome or acquiesce to obstacles/barriers (e.g. urging to attend rehabilitation, pushing at an optimal level)

weeks'), the athlete is likely to feel frustrated. This frustration stems from the mismatch in the type of support being provided and the support preferences of the athlete. Additionally, there is evidence that certain types of injuries tend to evoke the provision of certain forms of support. For example, tangible support, in the form of personal assistance, has been linked to the visibility and mobility of the injured athlete.[12] Remember, however, just because certain types of injuries are more likely to elicit certain types of support, it does not mean that this is the type of support preferred by injured athletes.

The right amount of support

For social support to be most useful, it must be provided in the right quantity or amount. Incongruencies may occur when the amount of support provided exceeds the recipient's expectations or desires.[5] For instance, athletes often have deeply ingrained norms of physical independence. Thus, when a family member offers physical assistance to an injured athlete, it may be rejected because the athlete views that assistance as coddling or doting. Indeed, these norms about the appropriate amount of attention that injured athletes should receive may be more entrenched in certain sports (e.g., wrestling) and may influence the degree to which athletes even seek medical care.[13]

Alternatively, problems may occur when recipients' expectations or needs exceed the amount of support made available by support providers. Research with individuals who were hospitalized for severe injuries and illnesses found that they reported a gradual but significant decline in perceived social support.[14] Similarly, athletes who experience severe or long-standing injuries may find that their social networks deteriorate or become strained over time. For instance, following an injury, athletes often feel that they have been 'shelved' or 'forgotten' by their coaches and teammates once they are no longer 'producing' in the athletic realm. This is illustrated in the following quotes from an elite skier who experienced a season-ending injury:

> I felt shut up, cut off from the whole ski team. That was one of the problems I had. I didn't feel like I was being cared for ... Once I got home, it was like they [the ski team] dropped me off at home, threw all my luggage in the house and were like 'See you when you get done.' I had a real, real hard time with that because I didn't want to feel cut off from the whole team. (See ref. 15, pp 369–70 therein.)

The right time for the support

The timing of the support that is provided is another significant factor when considering the effectiveness of social support. We know that the way individuals cope with stress can change over time. In the context of athletic injuries, shortly after an injury, athletes may prefer esteem/emotional support. Over time, as injured athletes receive medical care and come to understand the nature and extent of their injuries, there may be a preference for more informational social support.[12] Based on the above, those in contact with injured athletes must be astute observers/listeners of how support preferences of injured athletes may change and, when possible, match this to the type of support that is being provided.

Conclusions regarding the optimal matching framework

To conclude, the optimal support framework asserts that for social support to function adequately the 'right type' of support must be provided, in the 'right amount', and at the 'right time'. Given these complexities, it is not so surprising that occasional problems occur during the social exchange process between injured athletes, significant others, and medical professionals.

Role of significant others: family members, coaches, and teammates

This section focuses on the role that various significant others (family members, coaches, and teammates) play relative to the injured athlete. This discussion includes a summary of what types of social support injured athletes tend to expect from these people, as well what the research has indicated about the injured athletes' satisfaction with the providers.

Family members

Family members are a vital part of the injured athletes' social network and are often the only support providers that have been through all facets of the injury with the athlete. In the case of chronic, particularly severe, or difficult to diagnose injuries, family members may be especially prone to feeling emotionally overextended and frustrated. When medical professionals are working with family members under these circumstances, it is especially significant to acknowledge the family member's sustained efforts.

There are several characteristics of the injured athlete–family member relationship that bear mentioning. First, it is clear that injured athletes rely on family members for several types of support, including esteem/emotional, tangible, and motivational, and to a lesser extent informational support.[11,16] Thus, when working with the injured athlete's family, the medical professional will do well to inform them of the diverse role they will likely play in supporting the injured athlete.

Second, although family members play a variety of supporting roles for the injured athlete, the provision of esteem/emotional support seems to be one of the more critical forms of support. In one study, the family members were frequently described by injured athletes through statements such as: 'my parents were really there for me,' 'they didn't help in a direct way, just being there,' and 'understood what it would mean to me to be back [to competitive sport]'.[16]

Finally, injured athletes have tended to report relatively high levels of satisfaction with the support that family members and their spouse/partners provide,[11,16] with one study showing that spouses/partners were viewed as having a positive influence in over 90% of the cases.[11] This may be because family members are one of the support providers who tend to view their role largely as that of providing unconditional support and acceptance of the injured athlete.

Coaches

The role that coaches can play relative to the injured athletes' successful recovery is both complex and unique. Coaches play a potentially vital role in keeping athletes involved in the team throughout an injury and in terms of helping injured athletes make a successful transition from rehabilitation back into sport.

Despite the importance of the coach's role relative to social support for the injured athlete, there is evidence that the coach–injured athlete relationship is one that injured athletes are more likely to view ambivalently or negatively.[11,16] Although this pattern of results probably occurs for myriad reasons, it most often seems to be a function of the somewhat 'conditional' nature of the coach–athlete relationship. That is, when an athlete 'goes out' with an injury, coaches still have responsibilities to the remainder of their team and may have limited time to devote to the injured athlete. Additionally, the informal nature of many team settings may prevent some injured athletes from seeing the coach–athlete relationship as a true 'work' relationship. As described by one athlete:

I think when I came back from my knee injury he [my coach] kind of turned toward the other athletes because he knew I wasn't going to be the girl who was going to get him results that season. That really hurt me. That was the thing that really crushed me. (See ref. 16, pp. 384–5 therein.)

Teammates

The role that teammates and team captains can play relative to injured athletes can vary from minimal to profound. That is, in some cases, when athletes are injured they expect and receive little in terms of support from their teammates. The role of teammates seems to be influenced by a variety of factors including: time of the injury in relation to the competitive season (e.g., injury occurs during the off-season versus mid-season), the length of time the team has been together (e.g., newly formed versus long-standing social contact among team members), and gender (e.g., female athletes may prefer greater amounts of contact with teammates as compared to males).

It appears that, similar to family members, teammates can be an important source of several types of social support (i.e., esteem/emotional, informational, tangible, and motivational).[11] However, several areas may present difficulties for the injured athlete–teammate relationship. First, it can be difficult for injured athletes to watch other teammates or athletes replace them during their injury, and possibly permanently. As professional race-car driver, Ernie Irvan, noted, 'A racer's greatest fear is not perishing in one of these race cars. It's being injured and having to watch someone else drive his car.' (ref. 17, p. 47 therein). The issue of being replaced may be especially sensitive and relevant prior to major competitions. Naturally, most athletes want to be a part of major competitions, so watching athletes do what the injured athlete would desperately like to be doing can be difficult. Additionally, in the months before major competitions, athletes often step up their level of training. This boost in training intensity can increase the disparity between the injured athlete's and the replacement athlete's level of play, thereby decreasing the chance the injured athlete will be able to regain his/her spot post-injury.

A second potential difficulty in the relationship between injured athletes and teammates is likely to occur when a high-profile injured athlete returns to competition and draws a great deal of media and fan attention. For example, in the early 1990s, the professional athlete Bo Jackson was prominently featured in the media for not only his athletic accomplishments but also his phenomenal recovery from major surgery. Jackson, now retired from concurrent careers in US professional football *and* baseball leagues, had his career interrupted when he had surgery to fit an artificial hip replacement. When Jackson returned to professional baseball some of his teammates—who had been working hard in his absence—grew weary of all the attention Jackson received. The media surrounded one of Jackson's teammates after Jackson's first game back and asked him what he thought of Jackson's comeback. His teammate replied, 'I don't want to be smart, but don't ask me about Bo Jackson. We just won a big game, OK? Let's talk about tonight's game.'[18] Another teammate was overheard grumbling, 'Isn't there anyone else on this team?' (See ref. 18, p. 24 therein.) In short, the relationship between injured athletes and their teammates can be positive and supportive, but the competition between teammates can also resemble the interactions found in classic sibling rivalry.

The effects of social support

What influence, if any, do significant others have on an injured athlete, relative to outcomes such as athletes': (1) short-term, postinjury emotional adjustment, and (2) rehabilitation adherence and recovery? These issues are discussed in the following section.

Postinjury adjustment

Outside of the realm of sport, numerous studies have found that individuals who report higher levels of social support tend to report higher levels of emotional adjustment when coping with health-related stressors.[19] Within the sport realm, a survey of athletic trainers indicated that athletes who had high social support were more likely to cope successfully with their rehabilitation.[20] There are a variety of reasons why individuals with high levels of social support seem to fare better psychologically when coping with health-related stressors. First, these individuals may feel they have someone who will listen to their concerns. Thus, significant others serve as an emotional outlet for those experiencing health-related stress. This view is illustrated in the statement from a male athlete who had experienced a season-ending injury but who had a strong social support system. He noted:

> I was emotional. I needed to get a good cry out every week. So, every Saturday, I'd sit down with a good friend of mine and get my tears out and everything like that—it was something that I needed to do.[1]

Additional ways that social support may facilitate the psychological adjustment of injured athletes is through the information that is communicated about the nature of the health stressor. When individuals receive information about what to expect about their health status, it can relieve their anxiety and feelings of uncertainty. This information can be especially useful when it comes from a high status support such as a team captain or close friend. Again, in the words of the same athlete noted above:

> My friends [teammates who have had the same injury] are kind of a resource. So, I saw what they did when they blew out their knee. And I asked them a lot of questions before I had surgery, about what to do. But after that [surgery], I also used them for support ... 'How should my knee be feeling in

certain situations? What I should I be doing? What were they doing as far as certain activities?' So I use those guys as buddies, give them a good hug and what not, but also for really good technical knowledge.[1]

Finally, the motivational factors of social support are also thought to facilitate psychological functioning and lift the feelings of depression that often follow a severe injury. As noted by one elite skier:

It really helps being around people [other injured athletes] that can push you...For me that was a huge part...I'd never been really all that aggressive with my physical training before my injury and now I am. It's something new for me and I needed that motivation.[1]

Adherence and recovery

Are injured athletes' adherence, and in turn, recovery levels influenced by their social networks? In general, we know that individuals have difficulty initiating or modifying behaviors if there is no concomitant support from their environment. Because a significant portion of both our identity and our behavior is socially defined and reinforced,[21] we need to examine the social context of health outcomes such as adherence. The role of social support on rehabilitation adherence has been examined in a variety of studies.[22–25] This research has not produced uniform results with respect to the role of social influence, i.e., some studies have indicated that social support does have a significant influence on rehabilitation adherence and other studies have suggested it does not. This pattern of results seems to be related to the way that social support has been measured. In particular, it appears that when social support for rehabilitation is measured there is a more consistent relationship between social support and rehabilitation adherence.[24,25] However, when global measures of social support are used, the relationship between social support and adherence tends not to emerge as significant.[22]

What implications does the above have for medical practitioners? It suggests that, for example, an injured athlete's family may be emotionally supportive of the injured athlete but may not, for example, be able to transport the athlete to rehabilitation sessions (perhaps because the family does not really want the athlete to return to competitive sport or the family has other commitments or pressures). This type of situation will likely be problematic in terms of the athlete's adherence levels. In one clinical case I observed, a physiotherapist noticed that an injured high-school athlete was attending few rehabilitation sessions because of his parents' work schedules and the athlete's inability to drive himself to rehabilitation. The physiotherapist arranged for a teammate/close friend of the athlete to bring him to his rehabilitation sessions. In exchange for this assistance, the teammate was permitted to use some of the weight equipment in the rehabilitation center, which in turn allowed the teammate and the injured athlete to work out together.

Strategies for communicating with significant others

The discussion thus far has focused on defining social support and reviewing its influence. The remainder of this chapter will highlight strategies that can be used to facilitate communication between the medical practitioner and coaches, family members, and teammates.

Be patient

When athletes are injured their sense of identity, belonging, and sometimes their professional livelihood can be challenged.[26] But the psychological stress that often accompanies an injury can extend beyond the athlete. For instance, teammates and coaches of the injured athlete may perceive their own athletic aspirations have been thwarted by the injury if the injured athlete was a key contributor to their team and/or the injury occurred during an important time of the season. Coaches may experience guilt if they thought that they could have prevented the injury through alternative training practices. Parents may experience grief at the sudden loss of health they see in their son/daughter. Consequently, athletes' significant others may not always be at their 'interpersonal best' following an injury. Sometimes the medical practitioner is well advised simply to 'be patient' with athletes' significant others and not take their outbursts and impatience personally. Usually, the negative emotions of the support providers are aimed at the situation (e.g., loss of opportunities) rather than at the medical practitioner.

Be a patient advocate

For a variety of reasons, injured athletes may be the recipients of 'confusing' social support from significant others (e.g., family members, coaches, teammates). For instance, the team culture of some sports seems to support athletes' continued participation despite significant injuries. This type of attitude is reflected in team slogans such as 'no pain, no gain', 'pain don't hurt', and 'there are no injuries on Super Bowl Sunday'. These views towards injuries may be particularly salient in contact sports and/or sports which reinforce traditional views of masculinity, identity, and character development (see ref. 13 for a review). As more women enter competitive sports, however, the extent to which they are socialized to accept 'giving up their body' for sport is evident.

Another factor that may contribute to the ambivalent nature of social support that injured athletes receive is because many sports are considerably more competitive than they were a decade ago and, consequently, there is more at stake in terms of athletic scholarships and sponsorships. In some instances, this growing professionalization of sport has resulted in situations where parents may provide subtle encouragement for injured athletes to return to play before they are psychologically or physically ready.[27] Finally, due the competitive pressure they are under, coaches may also rush athletes to return to competitive participation prematurely.[28] One study compared the criteria that coaches and medical professionals used in evaluating athletes' readiness to return to competition.[29] Researchers found that coaches were likely to use the game criticality (e.g., close versus one-sided game) and player status (e.g., starter versus non-starter) as relevant factors in the decision-making process relative to an athlete's return to competition. In contrast, medical personnel did not view the above factors as relevant considerations and were more likely to consider the extent to which the athlete had physically recovered. To summarize, the medical practitioner should recognize that an athlete's social networks are not necessarily aligned with promoting the best interests of the injured athlete.

Based on the above, the medical practitioner should be prepared to clearly state under what conditions the injured athlete will receive clearance for returning to practice and/or competition. The need for this type of clear and direct communication may be particularly warranted in those circumstances in which the injured athlete is a minor and is less able to negotiate an appropriate outcome on his/her own behalf.[27]

Encourage significant others to demonstrate acceptance of and build confidence in injured athletes

A common challenge for injured athletes is how to overcome their loss of self-confidence and/or a fear of reinjury. This fear of reinjury or loss of self-confidence can be particularly arresting among athletes who participate in high-risk sports. In the end, it is the athletes themselves who must employ strategies to regain their self-confidence. There are, however, ways in which support providers can communicate their acceptance and support of athletes during this process. Let's look at an example of a positive coach–athlete relationship that illustrates this point.

Top-notch diver Greg Louganis, hit his head on the diving board during a preliminary round of the 1988 Olympics. Louganis still had to complete several more dives to remain in the competition. Under these conditions, many athletes would have experienced a significant loss of self-confidence and would have withdrawn from the competition entirely or opted to 'play it safe' on the remaining dive(s). During the time between dives, Louganis' coach, Ron O'Brien, provided Louganis with some vital and well-timed social support to boost his self-confidence. First, O'Brien told him, 'You don't have to do this. You don't have to do anything. No matter what you decide, I'm behind you 100%' (see ref. 30, p. 8 therein). In this way, O'Brien demonstrated a tremendously powerful form of support—that of unconditional support and acceptance.

Once Louganis decided to remain in the competition, O'Brien told Louganis 'You've done this [the upcoming dive] a thousand times in practice, just do like you do it' (see ref. 30, p. 9 therein). Thus, O'Brien was reminding Louganis that he had a long, successful track record of executing the dive. Interestingly, the approach that O'Brien used is very closely aligned with what the research would suggest. Specifically, it has been shown that one of the most important sources of self-confidence is successful past experiences.[31] Thus, if significant others want to be 'supportive' of injured athletes who are experiencing a loss of self-confidence, one of the most potent ways of doing this is to structure the environment in such a way that athletes have meaningful (i.e. not too easy) successes. Once athletes have had these successes, significant others may also need to remind that athlete of these successes—just as O'Brien did for Louganis. In the case of Louganis, he was able to overcome his fear, continue to dive, and win a gold medal in his event.

Work with significant others to avoid the out of sight/out of mind syndrome

As noted earlier, some athletes will find that their support networks deteriorate over time, and that this may be especially likely to happen among athletes who have experienced severe injuries. As Olympic ski racer Edith Thys noted about her injuries, 'Once out of the hospital, the trauma subsides, but so does the attention' (cited in ref. 32). Similarly, when American football standout, Jerry Rice, was out of competition with an extended injury his young son announced that, 'I want to play football this year and I want to be like J. J. Stokes' (the player who had replaced Rice in the line-up during his injury). Incredulous that their son didn't want to be like his father, his mother questioned him about his choice of role model. The son replied, matter-of-factly, 'J.J.'s catching the long ball and Dad isn't' (see ref. 33, p. 78 therein). In short, the attention given to the injured athlete is often fleeting.

In conclusion, based on both anecdotal as well as research evidence, there is a need for supportive environments to be maintained and sustained throughout the course of an athlete's injury. What are some specific strategies that can be used to accomplish this? Medical practitioners may encourage coaches and/or team captains to set up schedules for keeping in contact with injured athletes through weekly or monthly call sheets. These schedules can be used as reminders to maintain contact with athletes as well as recording comments or concerns that relate to athletes' injuries.

Another more preventive approach focuses on structuring the environment in such a way that injured athletes are not as likely to be 'out of sight' from significant others during their injuries. This type of approach is embedded in practices such as having injured athletes complete as much of their rehabilitation as possible in the presence of their team members. For instance, a basketball athlete recovering from a knee injury may need to use a stationary bike as part of his/her rehabilitation program. Under some circumstances, this activity can just as easily be completed in the gym while the rest of the team is practicing, as it is the athletic training room. One of the benefits of having the athlete complete rehabilitation in the presence of the rest of the team is that the athlete will typically feel more connected to the team, and it also means that the team can recognize and support the effort that the injured athlete is putting into rehabilitation.[32] For this type of approach to work effectively there must be open communication between medical professionals, the coaching staff, and the injured athlete.

References

1. Gould, D., Udry, E., Bridges, D., and Beck, L. (1996). Psychology of ski racing injuries. *Grant report to United States Olympic Committee*, pp. 203. USOC, Colorado Springs, CO.
2. Durkheim, E. (1952). *Suicide*. Free Press, New York.
3. Hardy, C. J. and Crace, R. K. (1993). The dimensions of social support when dealing with sport injuries. In *Psychological basis of sport injuries* (ed. D. Pargman), pp. 121–44. Fitness Information Technology, Morgantown.
4. Israel, B. and Schurman, S. (1990). Social support, control, and the stress process. In *Health behavior and health education* (ed. K. Glanz, F. Lewis, and B. Rimer), pp. 187–215. Jossey Bass, San Francisco, CA.
5. Shumaker, S. A. and Brownell, A. (1984). Toward a theory of social support: Closing conceptual gaps. *Journal of Social Issues*, **40**, 11–36.
6. Cutrona, C. E. and Russell, D. W. (1990). Type of social support and specific stress: toward a theory of optimal matching. In *Social support: an interactional view* (ed. B. Sarason, I. Sarason, and G. Pierce), pp. 319–66. Wiley, New York.
7. Thoits, P. A. (1986). Social support as coping assistance. *Journal of Consulting and Clinical Psychology*, **54**, 416–23.
8. Thoits, P. A. (1995). Stress, coping, and social support processes: Where are we? What next? *Journal of Health and Social Behavior*, (extra issue), 53–79.
9. Martin, R., Davis, G. M., Baron, R. S., Suls, J., and Blanchard, E. B. (1994). Specificity in social support: perceptions of helpful and unhelpful provider behaviors among irritable bowel syndrome, headache, and cancer patients. *Health Psychology*, **13**, 432–9.
10. Dakof, G. A. and Taylor, S. E. (1990). Victim's perceptions of social support: What is helpful from whom? *Journal of Personality and Social Psychology*, **58**, 80–9.
11. Udry, E. (1997). Support providers and injured athletes: A specificity approach. *A Journal of Applied Sport Psychology*, **9**, S34.
12. Johnston, L. (1998). The provision of social support to injured athletes: a qualitative analysis. *Journal of Sport Rehabilitation*, **7**, 267–84.
13. Wiese-Bjornstal, D. M., Smith, A. M., Shaffer, S. M., and Morrey, M. A. (1998). An integrated model of response to sport injury: Psychological and sociological dynamics. *Journal of Applied Sport Psychology*, **10**, 46–69.

14. Wilcox, V. L., Kasl, S. V., and Berkman, L. F. (1994). Social support and physical disability in older people after hospitalization: A prospective study. *Health Psychology*, **13**, 170–9.

15. Gould, D., Udry, E., Bridges, D., and Beck, L. (1997). Stress sources encountered when rehabilitating from season-ending ski injuries. *The Sport Psychologist*, **11**, 381–403.

16. Udry, E., Gould, D., Bridges, D., and Tuffey, S. (1997). People helping people? Examining the social ties of athletes coping with burnout and injury stress. *Journal of Sport and Exercise Psychology*, **19**, 369–95.

17. Hinton, E. (1995). Speedy recovery. *Sports Illustrated*, October 9, 46–7.

18. Verducci, T. (1993). Hip, hip, hooray. *Sports Illustrated*, May 15, 22–30.

19. Cohen, S. and Wills, T. A. (1985). Stress, social support, and the buffering hypothesis. *Psychological Bulletin*, **98**, 310–57.

20. Wiese, D., Weiss, M., and Yukelson, D. (1991). Sport psychology in the training room: A survey of athletic trainers. *The Sport Psychologist*, **5**, 15–24.

21. Brustad, R. J. and Ritter-Taylor, M. (1997). Applying social psychological perspectives to the sport psychology consulting process. *The Sport Psychologist*, **11**, 107–19.

22. Udry, E. (1997). Coping and social support among injured athletes following surgery. *Journal of Sport and Exercise Psychology*, **19**, 71–90.

23. Byerly, P. N., Worrell, T., Gahimer, J., and Domholdt, E. (1994). Rehabilitation compliance in an athletic training environment. *Journal of Athletic Training*, **29**, 352–5.

24. Duda, J. L., Smart, A. E., and Tappe, M. K. (1989). Predictors of adherence in the rehabilitation of athletic injuries: An application of personal investment theory. *Journal of Sport and Exercise Psychology*, **11**, 367–81.

25. Fisher, A. C., Domm, M. A., and Wuest, D. A. (1988). Adherence to sports-related rehabilitation programs. *Physician and Sportsmedicine*, **16**, 47–52.

26. Danish, S. (1986). Psychological aspects in the case and treatment of athletic injuries. In *Sport injuries: the unthwarted epidemic* (ed. P. Vinger, and E. Hoerner), pp. 345–53. PSG, Boston.

27. Heil, J. (1993). *Psychology of sport injury*. Human Kinetics, Champaign, IL.

28. Crossman, J. (1997). Psychological rehabilitation from sports injuries. *Sports Medicine*, **23**, 333–9.

29. Flint, F. A. and Weiss, M. R. (1992). Returning injured athletes to competition: A role and ethical dilemma. *Canadian Journal of Sport Sciences*, **17**, 34–40.

30. Louganis, G. and Marcus, E. (1995). *Breaking the surface*. Random House, New York.

31. Bandura, A. (1977). Self-efficacy: Toward a unifying theory of personality change. *Psychological Review*, **84**, 191–215.

32. Taylor, J. and Taylor, S. (1997). Psychological approaches to sports injury rehabilitation. Aspen, Gaithersburg, MD.

33. Silver, M. (1997). Final push. *Sports Illustrated*, December 15, 72–88.

9 *Returning to action and the prevention of future injury*

Mark B. Andersen

Once the initial shock of an athletic injury is over and the athlete has settled into a rehabilitation routine, the questions of returning to participation in sport and the prevention of future injuries loom larger and larger as recovery proceeds. Returning a recovering athlete to full sport participation is a complex and multifaceted process, which is influenced by a variety of factors that include the characteristics of the injury along with biological, psychological, and social variables. A biopsychosocial model of athletic injury rehabilitation has been developed (see Fig. 1.1),[1] which is helpful when considering preparing athletes to return to their sports in that it reminds practitioners of the large number of factors that influence the road to full recovery. Medical practitioners have a variety of standards to determine when an athlete might be ready to return (e.g., percentage of preinjury strength, laxity of joint, range of motion), but the picture of returning to sport covers a much broader canvas than physical and physiological recovery.

Characteristics of the injury

The type, course, severity, location, and history of an athletic injury all have an influence on the rehabilitation process. For example, if a runner fractures a thumb while trying to break a fall from being tripped, that location has much less dire consequences than a similar break in a big toe. The more 'central' the injury is to the sport performance (e.g., shoulder in swimming), the more likely the rehabilitation will be complex. If the body part in question is central to the athlete's sport, then the probability increases that the athlete will become anxious about reinjury, ruminate about not being able to come back 100% fit, and even withdraw from the sport. The severity of the injury will obviously influence the duration of rehabilitation and the percentage of recovery, but severity may also lead to psychosocial disruptions. If the injury is severe enough, the athlete may be in hospital or quite restricted in terms of movement. Such an injury may lead to isolation, in that the athlete cannot attend practice and team meetings. This isolation from coaches and team-mates represents a large withdrawal of social support, and social support is consistently shown to be positively related to health outcomes (see the section on Social/contextual factors below).

The history of the injury also has an influence on the response to rehabilitation and the prospects of returning to sport. If the injury is the first serious one an athlete has sustained, the initial response may be quite devastating. Athletes who are not accustomed to time off from their sports may find a first serious injury extremely disruptive to their daily lives, in that the routine of training has now disappeared. After the initial disruption of the injury for these first-timers, the athletes may, in their haste to get back to their sports, try to accelerate their recovery by doing more than is requested by medical practitioners. Motivation to perform rehabilitation exercises may not be much of a problem with first-time injured athletes, but holding them back from doing too much may be more of a concern. The dangerous more-is-better thinking, such as 'if 2 sets of 20 leg curls is good, then 4 sets must be twice as good', needs to be addressed early in the rehabilitation process to insure that athletes only do what is prescribed. Otherwise, athletes may set themselves at risk of retarding their rehabilitation by doing too much too soon.

For athletes who have had serious injuries before, the rehabilitation and return to sport may be a bit smoother in that they 'know the drill', are familiar with rehabilitation processes, and have already had the experience of returning successfully to sport. In other cases, however, if the second or third injury comes right on the heels of returning to full participation from a previous injury, then the athlete may be even more devastated than a first-timer, because all the hard work and pain of rehabilitation has been for nothing. Examining the history of the injury does not give us the whole picture, but it does offer clues and suggestions about how athletes may approach rehabilitation and how they may respond to the prospects of returning to sport. For example, if the athlete has gone through two knee reconstructions in the past, the trepidation and anxiety about getting back on the field and reinjuring a knee may be substantial. That anxiety may lead to heightened stress responsivity, and highly stressed people have a tendency to be more likely to incur injury.

Sociodemographic factors

These factors may have some influence on the course of rehabilitation and the readiness to return to sport. Age is an obvious factor in rehabilitation and healing. Younger athletes heal faster than older ones. The same sort of trauma for a 19-year-old athlete and a 45-year-old one will probably have substantially different time courses for recovery. The socioeconomic status of the athlete, especially if the sport is the major source of income (or future source of income), can have a profound effect on the rehabilitation process.

Financial concerns may push the athlete to return to sport too early or lead to the athlete denying pain in order to get the go-ahead to return. If sport is one's livelihood, then an injury is indeed quite threatening and anxiety provoking. Professional athletes, maybe even more than other athletes, need to have the intricacies, time lines, and progress markers of rehabilitation explained to them to ease their anxieties about their ability to earn a living and provide for their families. In a recent study, one of the most important things professional athletes wanted during rehabilitation was 'a realistic timeline for recovery'.[2] Professional athletes often felt they were pushed to come back too early, returning to the sport anxious about reinjury.

Gender and race/ethnicity also may influence injury rehabilitation and return to sport, but probably because of social and contextual factors (see below), rather than gender and ethnicity *per se.*

Biological factors

Biological factors play an obvious role in recovery and return to sport. If the athlete has seriously overtrained and is close to burnout when an injury occurs, then his/her resources, both psychological and physiological, will be depleted and thus recovery will be delayed. The overtrained athlete is not uncommon, and the injured overtrained athlete will start out the rehabilitation process at a distinct biological disadvantage.

An issue that arises in sports where eating disorders are common (gymnastics, diving, wrestling, figure skating) is nutrition. Proper nutrition is essential for rebuilding and repairing damaged tissue. For athletes with eating disorders, injuries are often caused, in part, by the sequelae of the disorder (weakened bones, higher fatigue). Also, when athletes with eating disorders stop exercise because of injuries, they may further decrease their food intake because of fears of gaining weight since they are no longer as physically active as they were before the injury. Their history of insufficient and poor nutrition leaves them with few resources for the recovery process. Helping injured athletes settle into healthy eating patterns, that will insure the proper intake of nutrients to aid the healing processes, is probably one of the areas that medical practitioners give limited attention to.

Sleep patterns may also be disrupted after an injury due to pain or anxieties about the injury and one's ability to come back. Inquiring about sleeping and eating patterns may help medical practitioners identify an appropriate intervention (e.g., pain management techniques to aid sleep) or whether to refer for expert consultation (e.g., to a nutritionist).

Psychological factors

Various psychological factors[3-8] affect the rehabilitation and return of injured athletes to full sport participation, including personality, how much they identify with the role of athlete, cognitive processes, emotional responses to rehabilitation and coming back (e.g., fear of reinjury), and behavioral patterns (e.g., adherence to rehabilitation exercise protocols). Personality factors may help or hinder the process of returning to play. For example, many elite athletes are highly dedicated, and, some might say, subclinically obsessive–compulsive about their training and competition. That dedication, for some, can be valuable during the rehabilitation process in that the athlete may adhere religiously to rehabilitation exercises. In other cases, that dedication to sport is part of an exclusive and foreclosed identity of self as athlete. For the athlete whose identity revolves almost exclusively around 'being an athlete', an injury poses a grave threat to one's sense of self. Researchers have found that those who identify most with the athlete role are also the ones more likely to experience psychological distress (depressed mood or even depressive episodes) when injured.[9–11] Injury brings up existential questions for these athletes ('Who am I, if I am not an athlete?'). A foreclosed athletic identity may result in a serious double-bind with injured athletes. The injured athlete wants desperately to return to play because that is what identity is all about, but there are also fears that the level of play one returns to will be lower than preinjury levels. The fears of returning in a 'diminished' capacity are again fears about identity. The thinking processes of an identity foreclosed athlete are often 'black and white' such as 'If I can't come back 100%, then I don't want to come back at all. It just isn't me.' This sort of irrational thinking sets the athlete up for negative emotional reactions upon returning to sport when (inevitably, in many cases) the standard of performance is not up to previous levels. If the negative emotional reaction is severe, and depression sets in, then it is probably time to refer to a sport or clinical psychologist.[12–14] Referral is a complex and delicate process, but a detailed examination of this topic is beyond the scope of this chapter. There will, however, be some suggestions as to 'when' and 'how' to start referral processes. There are also several good sources in the sport psychology literature for more information on the referral of athletes to mental health professionals.[15–17]

Anxiety about return comes from a variety of sources, such as the worry about not going back 100% as mentioned above. The prime source of anxiety in many cases is about the fear of reinjury, a fear that if not managed can actually increase the likelihood of a reinjury. There are many treatments for anxiety including psychopharmacological means (anxiolytic drugs), but taking mild tranquilizers is not usually an option for athletes on the road back to participation. There are, however, psychological skills such as relaxation, autogenic training, and systematic desensitization that are all aimed at anxiety responses, and several researchers have suggested that knowledge of these interventions become part of sport medical practitioner training.[2, 19–23] (For further information refer to Chapter 7.) The main behavior that most rehabilitation specialists are interested in is whether the athlete adheres to the prescribed exercises.[24] What is going to keep the athlete's behavior on track for recovery and return? The answer to that question lies at the heart of the Social/contextual factors box (see Fig. 1.2).

Social and contextual factors

Social and contextual factors concern the individual biology and psychology of the injured athlete and how these factors interact with the world around the athlete. For example, the quality and extent of one's social network, usually called social support, has been shown over and over again to have a substantial influence on injury resiliency[25] and on recovery from illness and surgery. An athlete has several levels of social support (e.g., family, peers, teammates and coaches, sports medicine team), and the quality of that support can have an impact on recovery and how the athlete feels about returning to play. For example, if the athlete has strong support from the coach and teammates, has been kept involved with the team (attends practices and team meetings), and is not pressured to come back too early (not an uncommon situation), then the athlete may feel more confident and supported in returning to play. In contrast, if the athlete has been isolated from the team, and knows other athletes have stepped into his/her role, then the athlete might feel pressured and anxious about coming back. Recent studies have shown that athletes want support from both the coach and teammates when in rehabilitation.[2]

In another important social situation, studies have repeatedly shown that social interactions with the medical practitioners rank the highest in what athletes consider to be important characteristics of helping professionals. Athletes want an honest and open communication style, and generally, a quality bedside manner from their physiotherapists and trainers. They want to be informed, and they want realistic timelines for recovery.[2] In all helping professions, the quality of the relationship between the caregiver and the receiver of care has a profound influence on health outcome. And this intimate form of social support from medical personnel can have a salubrious effect on athletes recovering from injury.

Questions of social/contextual factors revolve around conditions such as relationships with family, teammates, coaches, medical and psychological support, the other life stressors in the athlete's life (e.g., just moved to play in a new city), the environment of the sports medicine clinic, and whether sport is a major source of income. During the course of treatment, rehabilitation experts who deliver service to athletes might want to make inquiries as to how things are going in other aspects of the athletes' lives, to determine if some non-medical interventions may help the rehabilitation process along. Something as simple as talking to the coach and helping out on the sidelines by recording statistics during practice may significantly improve an athlete's mood and motivation to complete the rehabilitation exercises.[26]

Intermediate biopyschological outcome

The Intermediate Biopsychological Outcomes box (in Fig. 1.2) contains the variables (range of motion, limb strength, joint laxity, etc.) by which one can chart the recovery process. Signs of no, or slower than expected improvement in any of these variables would be a red flag that something is not going according to plan. The most subjective factors are pain and affect. As with everything, pain occurs in a context, and pain tolerance can vary with motivation. If there is pain in joints or muscles long past a reasonable healing time, then there may be social or psychological conditions that help pain persist. If such a condition is present, about the worst thing a medical practitioner can say is: 'I think it's in your head, and I would like you to see a psychologist'. Such a statement serves the caregiver's needs ('I can't figure out what is wrong, so I am going to blame you'), and is usually alienating and counterproductive. Referral of the athlete to a behavioral specialist, such as a rehabilitation psychologist, is probably a good idea when no physical or physiological problem can account for poor recovery progress, but such a referral can be handled in a more appropriate manner than in the style illustrated above. For example, the practitioner could say to the athlete in a gentle manner: 'I am not sure why you still have so much pain. Sometimes athletes don't heal as fast as we [medical practitioners] think they should because they have a lot of other worries and concerns and stresses in their lives. And we know stress slows the healing process. I know you're probably worried about ..., so what I do in these types of situations is that I suggest we talk to our sport psychologist. He/she has helped a lot of athletes get a handle on the stressors in their lives.' Athletes may be wary of seeing a psychologist,[27,28] but this manner of talking to the athlete helps to demystify the psychological profession and normalizes seeing a mental health practitioner.[16,17]

Knowing when to refer an athlete to a counselor or psychologist depends on the medical practitioner's knowledge of the psychological sequelae of injury and the ability to identify the symptoms of psychological distress. For example, if practitioners are not sensitive to subtle signs of depression (some are, some aren't), then they won't 'know' that a referral is appropriate and necessary. Any maladaptive response to injury (identity crisis, substance abuse, depression) could be a reason for referral, but a practitioner needs to be sensitive to behavioral, cognitive, and affective responses to injury. Recognizing a broken finger is a relatively easy diagnosis to make for most medical practitioners working with athletes. Recognizing a broken spirit may be a bit more difficult.

The other subjective variable is affect. Displays of lowered or depressed affect in the clinic when doing exercises often means an athlete is not engaged in the recovery process. Such athletes may be doing their exercises half-heartedly. The athlete may be depressed or resigned to the probable end of a career. The athlete who is motivated, working hard, and smiling through the pain is not the one medical practitioners have to worry about. If the practitioner cannot discover the source of the disturbed affect and low motivational state, referral may be the best option for an athlete who is not progressing and who is not engaged in the recovery process.[16,17]

Rehabilitation outcome

The final box, Sport Injury Rehabilitation Outcomes (see Fig. 1.2), is where medical practitioners want the athlete to arrive after rehabilitation: fully functional, loving life, happy with treatment, and ready to return to sport. As one can see from the model, the number of variables that directly and indirectly influence these ultimate outcomes is staggering. This model illustrates that no matter how complex something like rehabilitation is, when looked at closely it becomes even more complex and convoluted. No one person can have the expertise to monitor all these variables. The model provides a sound basis for the formation of rehabilitation teams.[29–31] The teams could be composed of physicians, physiotherapists, athletic trainers, coaches (monitoring special exercises at practice for the recovering athlete), and teammates (e.g. stretching partner). Such an approach will provide the expertise and the social and emotional support that will best serve the athlete. Once the athlete is back on track we want them to stay injury-free, and some of the techniques used in rehabilitation can also be used for prevention.

The prevention of future injury

A theoretical interactional model of stress and athletic injury, which includes many psychosocial aspects that may influence injury outcome (e.g., personality, history of stressors, coping resources), has been developed.[32,33] At the heart of the model are the hypothesized mechanisms of the stress response that may increase the risk of athletic injury. When athletes are placed in potentially stressful athletic situations (e.g., returning to full play after recovering from an injury), they may experience a pronounced stress response. Stress responses contain cognitive, physical, physiological, perceptual, and attentional components that can predispose an athlete to injury. In terms of the athlete's cognitive appraisals of returning to competition, one athlete may appraise the situation as: 'This is great! It's good to be back. I am feeling strong, and I am going to whip some butt!' Another athlete may say: 'God, I hope I don't get injured again. Gee those guys look big. I don't see how I am going to get through this. Please coach, don't put me in.' The first athlete is having fun, and the stress response in this case is probably minimal. The second athlete is making cognitive appraisals that he/she does not really have the resources to cope with the demands of the situation and that the consequences of the situation could be dire. This highly anxious athlete would be having a substantial stress response.

Connected to negative cognitive appraisals of athletic situations are the physiological and attentional aspects of sympathetic activation that are most intimately connected to injury risk. When an athlete is under stress there is usually a generalized muscle tension (bracing). This tension sets up the athlete for injury in a variety of ways. The most obvious is that if one is fighting oneself through activating agonistic and antagonistic muscle groups, then one is moving tensely, landing awkwardly, not 'rolling with the punches,' and generally setting oneself up for a variety of musculoskeletal strains and sprains. Another way generalized muscle tension places one at risk of injury is through early fatigue onset. Playing tense through a whole soccer match depletes resources much faster than when playing loose and relaxed. Thus, the athlete becomes fatigued more quickly, and fatigue is a major culprit in the etiology of injury. Also, generalized muscle tension may interfere momentarily with generating a motor pattern that would help one get out of harm's way. For example, if a softball player is overly tense in the batter's box, not only will it be difficult to generate the motor pattern to swing at a ball in the strike zone, but that increased muscle tension may delay the execution of ducking when a wild pitch is coming at her head.

The attentional and perceptual changes associated with stress and which may contribute to injury risk involve peripheral narrowing and increased distractibility. Under stress, peripheral vision tends to narrow.[34] In many sports, having a wide field of vision is necessary for excellent play and for safety. For example, a quarterback in American and Canadian football needs to be able to read the field well to find receivers, but he also needs to be wary of tacklers coming in from the periphery. Detecting that one is about to be tackled lets one roll with that tackle. It is probably the undetected tackle that is more likely to result in injury.

Stress also causes one's attentional system to become more distractible. Such distractibility can lead to athletes focusing on task-irrelevant cues to the detriment of performance. For some athletes returning to sport after an injury, their own negative thinking (e.g., 'I hope I don't tweak this hammy again.') actually distracts them from the task at hand, and, thus, the task may be performed awkwardly, and injury may result. Another example of distractibility is during a gymnastics competition: one athlete may just be preparing for a complicated dismount when another athlete falls off a piece of apparatus in another part of the venue. The whole crowd goes 'Ohhhhhh' just as the athlete releases, so that the athlete's attention is pulled off-task by the crowd, he/she loses orientation, and lands dangerously.

One technique to lessen distractibility and improve concentration is distraction desensitization. The idea is based on the principle of habituation. In practice, the coach, assistant coach, or sport psychologist can introduce and slowly increase distracting stimuli. As athletes become habituated to one level or type of distracter, higher levels and different types of distracters are introduced, and then athletes become habituated to those, and so it goes until athletes can perform with bombs going off around them. Some coaches have been known to play rival teams' fight songs at high volume during practice so that the acoustic environment is familiar when they play the rival teams. As stated earlier, the ability to stay focused on the task at hand is central for injury prevention (in many areas besides sport, such as driving a car), and distraction desensitization is one method to use for aiding the concentration necessary for good (and safe) performance. Many other cognitive (e.g. thought-stopping, cognitive restructuring) and physiological/attentional interventions (e.g. relaxation, imagery) have been shown to lower stress and injury risk.[35–39] (For further information on these topics, refer to Chapter 7.)

Lessons learned

There are many lessons to take away from examining the variables that lead to readiness (or lack of thereof) to return to participation and the interventions that may increase resiliency to future injury. A central feature to understanding emotional and behavioral responses to injury and rehabilitation is the question of athletic identity.[40] Generally, those athletes whose self-image includes much more than what they do in their sports will have an easier time during recovery and return to sport than those who have foreclosed their athletic identity. For athletes with strong negative reactions (e.g., depression, radical mood swings, withdrawal) to injury, referral to a sport psychologist may be helpful and allow the foreclosed athlete to begin to identify and explore other aspects of self than being only an athlete. A central lesson here is to become sensitive to the cognitive, behavioral, and affective signs that the athlete is in some kind of psychological distress. The lesson to take away is that rehabilitation is a complex combination of biological, psychological, and social/environmental processes. Helping an athlete prepare to return to full participation is the ultimate goal of rehabilitation. In a true sense, all of athletic injury rehabilitation is made up of gradual steps to enable return to play, and intervention at any of the biopsychosocial levels may help to smooth the progression of recovery and return and act as prophylaxis to reduce the risk of future injury.

The lessons for preventing future injury obviously start with the basics of getting the athlete on a regular program of gradual warm-up and extensive stretching (along with other modified exercises) before practice, accompanied by cool-down and more stretching exercises after practice. Probably in both cases (before and after practice), these activities will require more time than they would if the athlete was not recovering from a recent injury.

Finally, working on the anxieties and maladaptive perceptions athletes have about return to participation, through psychological interventions (e.g., relaxation, cognitive restructuring), may lower stress responsivity and increase injury resiliency.

References

1. Brewer, B. W., Andersen, M. B., and Van Raalte, J. L. Psychological aspects of injury rehabilitation: Toward a biopsychosocial approach. In *Medical aspects of sport and exercise* (ed. D. I. Mostofsky and L. Zaichkowsky). Fitness Information Technology, Morgantown, WV. (In press.)
2. Francis, S. R., Andersen, M. B., and Maley, P. (2000). Physiotherapists' and male professional athletes' views of psychological skills for rehabilitation. *Journal of Science and Medicine in Sport*, 3, 17–29.
3. Latuda, L. (1995). The use of psychological skills in enhancing the rehabilitation of injured athletes. *Journal of Sport and Exercise Psychology*, 17, 70.
4. Ross, M. J. and Berger, R. S. (1996). Effects of stress inoculation on athletes' postsurgical pain and rehabilitation after orthopedic injury. *Journal of Consulting and Clinical Psychology*, 64, 406–10.
5. Smith, A. M., Scott, S. G. O., Fallon, W. M., and Young, M. L. (1990). Emotional responses of athletes to injury. *Mayo Clinic Proceedings*, 65, 38–50.
6. Taylor, A. H. and May, S. (1996). Threat and coping appraisal as determinants of compliance to sports injury rehabilitation: an application of protection motivation theory. *Journal of Sports Sciences*, 14, 471–82.
7. Theodorakis, Y., Beneca A., Malliou, P., and Goudas, M. (1997). Examining psychological factors during injury rehabilitation. *Journal of Sport Rehabilitation*, 6, 355–63.
8. Uemukai, K. (June, 1993). Affective responses and the changes in athletes due to injury. In *Proceedings of the 8th World Congress of Sport Psychology* (ed. S. Serpa, J. Alves, V. Ferreira, and A. Paula-Brito), pp. 500–3. International Society of Sport Psychology, Lisbon, Portugal.
9. Brewer, B. W. (1993). Self-identity and specific vulnerability to depressed mood. *Journal of Personality*, 61, 343–64.
10. Lavallee, D., Grove, J. R., Gordon, S., and Ford, I. W. (1998). The experience of loss in sport. In *Perspectives on loss: a sourcebook* (ed. J. H. Harvey), pp. 241–52. Brunner/Mazel, Philadelphia, PA.
11. Murphy, G. M., Petitpas, A. J., and Brewer, B. W. (1996). Identity foreclosure, athletic identity, and career maturity in intercollegiate athletes. *The Sport Psychologist*, 10, 239–46.
12. Newcomer, R. R., Roh, J., Perna, F. M., and Etzel, E. F. (1998). Injury as a traumatic experience: intrusive thoughts and avoidance behavior associated with injury among college student-athletes. *Journal of Applied Sport Psychology*, 10(Suppl.), S54. [Abstract]
13. Perna, F. M., Roh, J., Newcomer, R. R., and Etzel, E. F. (1998). Clinical depression among injured athletes: An empirical assessment. *Journal of Applied Sport Psychology*, 10, S54–S55. [Abstract]
14. Roh, J., Newcomer, R. R., Perna, F. M., and Etzel, E. F. (1998). Depressive

mood states among college athletes: Pre- and post-injury. *Journal of Applied Sport Psychology*, **10**(Suppl.), S54. [Abstract]

15. Andersen, M. B., Denson, E. L., Brewer, B. W., and Van Raalte, J. (1994). Disorders of personality and mood in athletes: Recognition and referal. *Journal of Applied Sport Psychology*, **6**, 168–84.

16. Heyman, S. R., and Andersen, M. B. (1998). When to refer athletes for counseling and psychotherapy. In *Applied sport psychology: personal growth to peak performance* (3rd edn) (ed. J. M. Williams), pp. 359–71. Mayfield, Mountain View, CA.

17. Van Raalte, J. L., and Andersen, M. B. (1996). Referral processes in sport Psychology. In *Exploring sport and exercise psychology* (ed. J. L. Van Raalte and B. W. Brewer), pp. 275–84. American Psychological Association, Washington DC.

18. Rotella, R. J. and Campbell, M. S. (1983). Systematic desensitization: Psychological rehabilitation of injured athletes. *Athletic Training*, **18**, 140–2, 151.

19. Ford, I. W. and Gordon, S. (1993). Social support and athletic injury: The perspective of sport physiotherapists. *Australian Journal of Science and Medicine in Sport*, **25**, 17–25.

20. Ford, I. W. and Gordon, S. (1997). Perspectives of sport physiotherapists on the frequency and significance of psychological factors in professional practice: Implications for curriculum design in professional training. *Australian Journal of Science and Medicine in Sport*, **29**, 34–40.

21. Ford, I. W. and Gordon, S. (1998). Perspectives of sport trainers and athletic therapists on the psychological content of their practice and training. *Journal of Sport Rehabilitation*, **7**, 79–94.

22. Gordon, S., Potter, M., and Ford, I. (1998). Toward a psychoeducational curriculum for training sport-injury rehabilitation personnel. *Journal of Applied Sport Psychology*, **10**, 140–56.

23. Wiese, D. M., Weiss, M. R., and Yukelson, D. P. (1991). Sport psychology in the training room: a survey of athletic trainers. *The Sport Psychologist*, **5**, 25–40.

24. Daly, J. M., Brewer, B. W., Van Raalte, J. L., Petitpas, A. J., and Sklar, J. H. (1995). Cognitive appraisal, emotional adjustment, and adherence to rehabilitation following knee surgery. *Journal of Sport Rehabilitation*, **4**, 23–30.

25. Hardy, C. J., Richman, J. M., and Rosenfeld, L. B. (1991). The role of social support in the life stress/injury relationship. *The Sport Psychologist*, **5**, 128–39.

26. Brewer, B. W., Petitpas, A. J., and Van Raalte, J. L. (1999). Referral of injured athletes for counseling and psychotherapy. In *Counseling in sports medicine* (ed. R. Ray and D. M. Wiese-Bjornstahl), pp. 127–41. Human Kinetics, Champaign, IL.

27. Linder, D. E., Brewer, B. W., Van Raalte, J. L., and DeLange, N. (1991). A negative halo for athletes who consult sport psychologists: Replication and extension. *Journal of Sport and Exercise Psychology*, **13**, 133–48.

28. Van Raalte, J. L., Brewer, B. W., Brewer, D. D., and Linder, D. E. (1992). NCAA Division II college football players' perceptions of an athlete who consults a sport psychologist. *Journal of Sport and Exercise Psychology*, **14**, 273–82.
29. Andersen, M. B. and Brewer, B. W. (1995). Organizational and psychological consultation in collegiate sports medicine groups. *Journal of American College Health*, **44**, 63–9.
30. Heil, J. (1993). Sport psychology, the athlete at risk, and the sports medicine team. In *Psychology of sport injury* (ed. J. Heil), pp. 1–13. Human Kinetics, Champaign, IL.
31. Wiese-Bjornstal, D. M. and Smith, A. M. (1993). Counseling strategies for enhanced recovery of injured athletes within a team approach. In *Psychological bases of sport injury* (ed. D. Pargman), pp. 149–82. Fitness Information Technology, Morgantown, WV.
32. Andersen, M. B., and Williams, J. M. (1988). A model of stress and athletic injury: Prediction and prevention. *Journal of Sport and Exercise Psychology*, **10**, 294–306.
33. Williams, J. M. and Andersen, M. B. (1998). Review and critique of the stress and injury model. *Journal of Applied Sport Psychology*, **10**, 6–25.
34. Andersen, M. B. and Williams, J. M. (1999). Athletic injury, psychosocial factors and changes during stress. *Journal of Sports Sciences*, **17**, 735–41.
35. Andersen, M. B. and Stoové, M. A. (1998). The sanctity of p < .05 obfuscates good stuff: A comment on Kerr and Goss. *Journal of Applied Sport Psychology*, **10**, 168–73.
36. Davis, J. O. (1991). Sports injuries and stress management: An opportunity for research. *The Sport Psychologist*, **5**, 175–82.
37. DeWitt, D. J. (1980). Cognitive and biofeedback training for stress reduction with university athletes. *Journal of Sport Psychology*, **2**, 288–94.
38. Kerr, G. and Goss, J. (1996). The effects of a stress management program on injuries and stress levels. *Journal of Applied Sport Psychology*, **8**, 109–17.
39. Ievleva, L. and Orlick, T. (1991). Mental links to enhanced healing: An exploratory study. *The Sport Psychologist*, **5**, 25–40.
40. Brewer, B. W., Van Raalte, J. L., and Linder, D. E. (1993). Athletic identity: Hercules' muscles or Achilles' heel? *International Journal of Sport Psychology*, **24**, 237–54.

10 *Developing a culture of change in the workplace: applying processes and principles from action research to sports injury settings*

David Gilbourne

Introduction

This chapter outlines how a process of systematic reflection can enhance working practice. The thinking behind a chapter of this nature is built around a series of intuitive connections. First of all, it is clear that all the chapters within this textbook are written with the sports medicine practitioner in mind. Second, it is likely that certain ideas and guidelines, embedded within the preceding chapters, will motivate practitioners to instigate 'changes' into their own working practice. It is proposed here that an awareness of certain action-research themes and processes might help to facilitate this process. In making the above observations there is no intention to suggest that, somehow, bringing about workplace change is straightforward. Clearly, changes in working practice can be assisted or limited by a number of factors such as the time and finance available, the capacity of existing facilities, and the available expertise. In addition, it is also possible that proposals for change may not be acceptable to all those who occupy the workplace. For all these reasons the introduction of new ideas can be a delicate and challenging process.

With the above caveats in mind, the present chapter is based upon the notion that formalized, ongoing, focused discussion allows current practice to be openly discussed and monitored. Central to this case is the term 'systematic' which, in turn, is associated with the view that clear, reflective procedures encourage a regular review of practice. In the following discussion such procedures draw on guidelines outlined primarily in the action-research literature.[1–6]

The idea of focusing on action research is associated with a feeling that research-based themes and processes can be transferred to non-research activity. The logic here is that action research, first and foremost, encourages reflection on practice. In a secondary sense, such reflection is intended to result in changes in working procedures. It seems fair to reason that the process of reflection would be helpful to medical practitioners whether research is taking place or not. So, whatever the motivation, be it the production of a research thesis or a straightforward desire to improve practice, reflection is seen to have a part to play. In this chapter, reflection is viewed as a process that can 'tap into' the creative capacity of practitioner groups and in doing so help them find their own solutions to their own problems. In addition, it is suggested that reflection might provide a platform from which practitioner groups decide how to integrate ideas from 'elsewhere' (i.e. from sport science). The bottom line is that reflection (of a systematic kind) can help practitioners improve practice in their own workplace.

The chapter has been divided into three sections. The first section introduces some of the theoretical issues which support the theme of reflection. In contrast, the second section outlines practical guidelines for undertaking systematic reflection. The final section has a more practical focus and reports on a 'reflective exercise' undertaken within a sports injury setting. This last section illustrates how an interdisciplinary group of sports medical practitioners participated in a systematic process of reflection and review in order to improve one aspect of their own working practice.

Action research and reflection: Establishing a theoretical platform

The topic of enhancing practice has received considerable attention from commentators who are interested in linking workplace change to the mechanism of reflection.[7,8] This same line of thinking has also led educationalists,[9] sport scientists,[10] and mixed cohorts of sport scientists and physiotherapists,[11] to ask similar questions through the application of action-research themes and processes.

Action research is associated with addressing practical problems in the workplace and encouraging practitioner groups to manage their own change in their own way.[1] This emphasis on 'action' is linked to the process of reflection.[1,9,15] More specifically, it is thought that reflection on current practice can stimulate debate amongst practitioner groups and so encourage adjustments and modifications to working procedures.[9] In all action-research projects this change process is framed within a cyclic model that includes a review of present practice, the subsequent planning for any change, the implementation and monitoring of that change, and (if necessary) further reflection and review (see Fig. 10.1). This procedural template helps to direct and set the tempo of any reflective project[11] and, in a general sense, this model, and variations of it, form the basis for contemporary action-research design.[1,4]

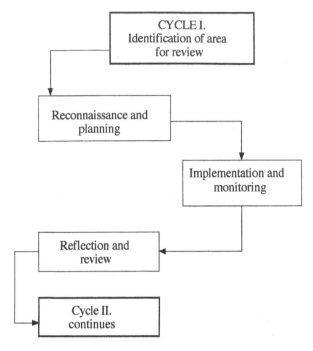

Fig. 10.1   The action research cycle.

The action-research literature has been influenced by the notion that there is a distinction between the 'certainties' of science and the 'swampy lowlands' which typify the reality of the workplace.[7,8] This line of thinking has led other commentators to link 'science-based' academic material with the terms 'professional knowledge' and 'craft knowledge' to describe the workplace-specific awareness developed by the practitioner.[9] The processes within action research have been devised to facilitate and monitor the blending of professional knowledge with established craft thinking.[9] In a similar way, the same processes have also been used to help practitioners develop and share craft knowledge.[9] With these aims in mind, action research has been used extensively within education[9,12] and healthcare settings.[13,14]

Within a sports injury setting, notions of craft and professional knowledge may be evident as the difference between a physiotherapist or athletic trainer understanding the theoretical concepts that underpin, for example, a goal-setting program, and his/her day-to-day capacity to engage injured athletes in the process.[10] Section three of the present chapter provides practical examples of how reflection encourages sports injury practitioners to 'grapple' with craft and professional knowledge issues.

In establishing a rationale for why reflection can enhance professional practice, a number of core messages have been emphasized. Sports injury practitioners (through the daily routine of practice in the workplace) develop a sense of 'craft' knowledge. Following on, reflection is presented as one process that can help practitioners 'get in touch' with their craft knowledge base. In addition, it is proposed that professional knowledge, typified by research output from academic institutions and other professional forums, can be integrated with craft knowledge and blended into the practice arena through the process of systematic reflection. More generally, this process has been linked to a cyclic model of reflection and action.

Practical guidelines for conducting systematic reflection

This second section outlines core strategies for the introduction and develop-ment of systematic reflection. The first set of guidelines relate to the role of a reflective 'facilitator'. When change is being undertaken in a systematic man-ner it is likely to be facilitated by a 'named' person. Although this role may be undertaken by an 'insider', it is also possible that someone from outside may be involved, for example from an academic institution or a consultancy firm. In the latter case, the process of reflection and change, be it driven by a research or a more practical agenda, may utilize an outside 'agent' to oversee matters.

It is important for whoever is facilitating a project for them to understand that organizing opportunities for groups to reflect is a core element of the cyclic structure.[15] The following guidelines refer to what different commen-tators have called a facilitator,[11] associate,[16] or consultant[17] and suggest that it is important:

- not to impose but to stimulate change;
- to focus primarily on establishing the process of reflection that leads to change;
- to facilitate/encourage practitioners to develop their own analysis of issues;
- to stress the notion of personal development.

In a more general sense, facilitating change might also require the person in the leadership role to:

- assist practitioners to monitor change by organizing reflective meetings and helping formally in the assessment of impact upon client groups.

It has already been noted that the process of ongoing reflection can be based around the action-research cycle outlined in Fig. 10.1. This will help to establish an organizational framework for 'steering' the reflective process. The cyclic framework also helps to set the tempo of reflection. These sentiments are supported by those who stress that participants in any reflective project should meet on a regular basis.[2,16]

This notion of maintaining a sense of 'tempo' is central to all reflective activity, as it is all too easy in the busy workplace to let the process fade away and allow day-to-day events to take priority over longer term development. With this in mind, the regular convening of 'reflective' groups becomes essential. These meetings provide an opportunity for practitioners to:

- generally reflect upon the impact of any ongoing changes;
- allow designated individuals to present feedback on specific issues (as illustrated in Section 3);
- make decisions about the way forward;
- identify how the changes will be monitored.

In addition to these procedural factors, a number of 'toolbox' items can help the reflective process to be effectively managed and monitored.[4] As well as suggesting the maintenance of a project file in which to collate materials such as agendas for meetings and action decisions, diary-keeping as an accompaniment to reflection is also emphasized.[4]

Maintaining a reflective diary can help those involved in a project to describe and capture those 'things' about practice that have occurred that day. Reflection is, therefore, formalized a little and this information can help to stimulate discussions at the meetings outlined earlier. The maintenance of a diary encourages the monitoring of your own performance and assists the evaluation of progress.[4]

These guidelines provide an outline structure for undertaking systematic reflection, and mirror elements of the practical illustration presented in the third section of this chapter. These ideas should be viewed flexibly, as different reflective projects are likely to adopt varying degrees of formality. For example, a research-driven project tends to signal outside involvement and a need for any monitoring to incorporate formal data-collection procedures. In contrast, a project developed 'intrinsically' within the workplace is unlikely to follow such a rigorous protocol.

Reflection in action

This final part of the chapter outlines a practical example of systematic reflection and collaboration.. 'I' (the author of this chapter) acted as the external facilitator of the project.

The following material is taken from an extended period of action-research in which I collaborated, for the most part, with sport physiotherapists. The primary focus of our work together was the athletes' sports injury experience.[18] Throughout this protracted exercise the workplace was a sports injury centre in the UK. During my time at this centre, a number of action research projects unfolded, and the process sketched out here involved practitioners from the disciplines of sports physiology (referred to throughout as sport scientists) and physiotherapy. The project aimed to monitor the early development of a change strategy that introduced body-fat measurement to injured athletes. This strategy formed part of a broader plan to share practice elements between staff who worked within the Sports-injury Rehabilitation Centre and an adjoining Human Performance Centre.

This story illustrates how a collaborative-reflective venture progressed within a sports injury setting, and allows aspects of the theoretical material, outlined in Section 1, to be viewed from an action perspective. The various components of reflection and action are presented as a series of collaborative phases (Fig. 10.2), in line with the structure outlined in Fig. 10.1. Insights into my 'external' facilitating role are provided by the inclusion of my own thoughts and observations. These personal reflections have been taken from my field diary, which helped me to keep a record of my role as a facilitator of the reflective process.

As highlighted in the second section, collaborative ventures can generate information from a number of sources, for instance observations, meetings, and interviews. Consequently, in addition to my own field notes, information generated by the members of the practitioner group is also presented. This material was recorded on audiotape and includes group meetings and one-to-one interviews between myself and the practitioners, and between myself and the injured athletes who attended the Centre.

Phase one: Starting the project

This particular project began when the chief physiotherapist at the Centre invited me to meet the staff and to present a case for starting an interdisciplinary reflective project, when I emphasized the benefits of reflective practice generally. Following a short discussion, the staff agreed that it would be valuable to monitor and reflect upon any changes currently taking place. The staff were also enthusiastic about exploring joint ventures between the rehabilitation and human performance arms of the Centre.

> It was clear that the sport scientists and physiotherapists saw value in cooperation and had a change of practice in mind. They had always seen a certain logic in the Rehabilitation and Human performance centre's linking expertise in some way and had in the past 'informally' cooperated in particular cases on such things as body-fat measurement. They were also keen to move this arrangement onto a more formal footing and saw developing the process of body-fat measurement as a logical first step. (Field notes.)

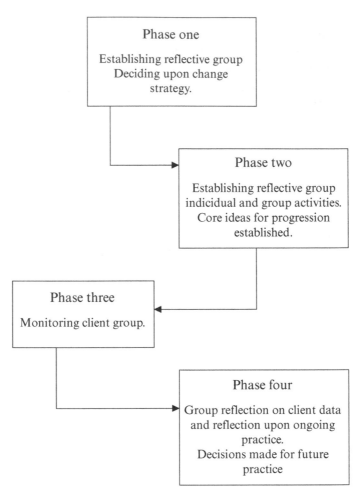

Fig. 10.2   Phases of reflection and collaboration.

With Fig. 10.1 in mind, I noted that the 'order' of the project was already out of sequence. It is normal practice to review practice carefully before moving towards the initiation of new ideas. In this case, however, the practitioners had already informally discussed the idea of introducing a body-fat measurement protocol (BFMP) into the Centre. Given such a background, it seemed reasonable to suppose that a form of spontaneous 'practitioner-led' review had already taken place.

> The group had in about 5 minutes agreed to liaise more and decided upon a change strategy. I was left to feel frustrated...the initial review cycle had seemingly been circumnavigated...this was hardly textbook stuff. For a while...driving home I was unsure about what had happened. 'So what'...I

thought, they had talked about change informally before and had decided to get on with it. I just needed to chase after them. (Field notes.)

Moments like these do highlight the realities of facilitating reflection in the 'real world'. The BFMP practice that had begun was based around a three-stage approach: initial education, measurement, and feedback. Initially, injured athletes attended a workshop on diet and body-fat issues at the Centre. This was followed by each athlete's body-fat being measured and the production (by the sport scientists) of a written report. After receiving the report, the players were given the option of discussing the findings at a further one-to-one meeting.

Phase two: Starting to reflect on action

To initiate the process of reflective practice as soon as possible, it was decided to convene a meeting to discuss what constitutes 'good practice', to review any body-fat procedures that had already been carried out, and to consider what the practitioners had hoped to achieve by introducing the BFMP. This group reflection process was preceded by the practitioners focusing on these issues during one-to-one semi-structured interviews.

The interview data was subjected to a coding analysis procedure, with the results being returned to all the practitioners prior to the next meeting. Providing feedback ahead of meetings helps to prime the reflection process.[18] In this sense, practitioners are able to reflect ahead of the meeting in which findings are typically reviewed in a more formal group setting.

A number of core themes emerged from the interviews (Fig. 10.3). Points 1–5 were associated with what was termed 'ideal practice'. The term 'ideal' was used as it was recognized that sometimes one-to-one contact was not always possible, that athletes may not always be totally committed to what sports science had to offer, and, finally, that at times the opportunity to review and monitor was limited.

In contrast, 'good practice' (points 6–10) constituted the practitioners' thoughts on the core elements that constitute sound professional conduct. Unlike the 'ideal' factors, these points were thought to be much more personally controllable.

The practitioners supported the development of the body-fat program (points 11–14) and made reference to intrinsic factors (such as the value to athletes) and to extrinsic issues (such as the procedure acting as a positive 'marketing' angle for the Rehabilitation centre). On a more cautious note, a number of concerns had already started to arise from the limited 'formalized' practice that had already taken place (points 15–17). For example, a debate on how best to start the process had already begun, and a need to identify the key educational elements of the process was also mentioned. The former I associated with a 'craft' knowledge issue; the latter more with the combined input of craft and professional knowledge.

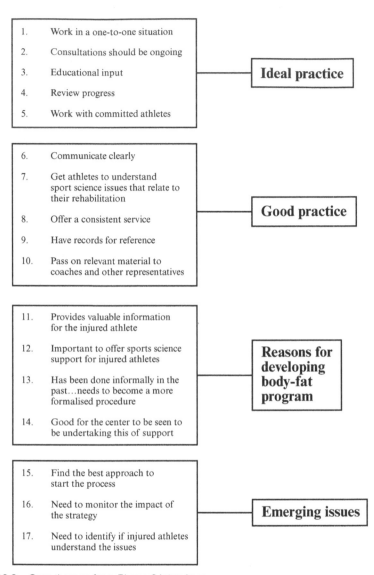

1.	Work in a one-to-one situation	
2.	Consultations should be ongoing	
3.	Educational input	**Ideal practice**
4.	Review progress	
5.	Work with committed athletes	

6.	Communicate clearly	
7.	Get athletes to understand sport science issues that relate to their rehabilitation	
8.	Offer a consistent service	**Good practice**
9.	Have records for reference	
10.	Pass on relevant material to coaches and other representatives	

11.	Provides valuable information for the injured athlete	
12.	Important to offer sports science support for injured athletes	**Reasons for developing body-fat program**
13.	Has been done informally in the past…needs to become a more formalised procedure	
14.	Good for the center to be seen to be undertaking this of support	

15.	Find the best approach to start the process	
16.	Need to monitor the impact of the strategy	**Emerging issues**
17.	Need to identify if injured athletes understand the issues	

Fig. 10.3 Core themes from Phase 2 interviews.

Reflection and review: An overview of the group meeting

The following material is taken from interview transcripts recorded during the first reflection meeting. Examples of dialogue between the practitioner group illustrate how the BFMP was reviewed and how ideas for change were explored. My role in this meeting was to help to facilitate dialogue and generally act as an informal chairperson.

During the meeting, the practitioners felt it was important to bring the body-fat procedure into line with points 1 and 3 of 'ideal practice'. For example, earlier interviews had indicated that one-to-one contact with athletes provided the ideal consultation format; monitoring an athlete's progress was also cited. The meeting initially discussed point 1, and reviewed the way one-to-one contact was occurring in the program. From this discussion, the practitioners voiced concerns that they might be forcing players to attend.

> ... if I'm constantly nagging them [the players] then it sometimes turns into a situation where they go along...because they've been nagged into it. (Reflection meeting transcript: sport scientist.)

Discussions of this nature encouraged the practitioners to focus on 'craft-based' procedural issues. In this context, one of the sport scientists responded by suggesting that non-attendance might also be worthy of discussion. I felt this comment reflected a wider group concern over the way the BFMP had been initially organized. As a result, it was suggested that some formal structuring of the post-measurement timetable could move the procedure forward in a positive manner.

> ... I wonder if there is a way round it. They may be thinking 'I don't want to waste our time' and therefore they haven't come back to follow it up. If we had a system, so rather than pushing the issues or not mentioning it again ... when we give them the report back we could also highlight time slots that are available during the week and if they want to they can sign up. (Reflection meeting transcript: sport scientist.)

The need to monitor the players was also mentioned:

> ...another thing that is interesting is how do we monitor [players] when we get them back in again. The only example so far is the tennis player. He felt he wasn't making any progress, but clearly the body fat showed that his body composition was changing. (Reflection meeting transcript: sport scientist.)

This aspect of the discussion highlighted the fact that some players with long-term injuries would return to the Centre for further treatment. In contrast, those with shorter term injuries might only be expected to visit the Centre once and often expect to be match-fit within a few weeks. The group felt that the measurement program could benefit both groups; however, it was also noted that longitudinal monitoring did provide the opportunity for the players to get ongoing feedback on body-fat progress.

> ... If you have got someone who is coming back you can basically measure the impact. If you have someone who is not coming back then you can't test them again. You can nevertheless pick-up something from them that indicates you have opened their eyes. (Reflection meeting transcript: sport scientist.)

The theme of monitoring was extended to encompass the need to understand how injured athletes were presently experiencing the measurement process:

Changes to present practice:

- build one-to-one meetings into the system
- move nearer to core components of 'ideal' practice

Decisions on monitoring procedures:

- seek athletes views on the body-fat program

Specifically to ascertain:

- how athletes view the issue of diet and sports injury
- if athletes understand the information they receive
- if athletes appreciate the process

Fig. 10.4   Core issues emerging from the Phase 2 group meeting.

...If we change now, we've changed it without really knowing why we have changed. (Reflection meeting transcript: sport scientist.)

Despite these final sentiments, some strategies for change did emerge from the meeting. Several core issues were identified, which formed the basis for moving the process forward (Fig. 10.4). Some factors required adjustments to be made to current practice, while others were associated with further strategies to help in the monitoring of practice. For example, one strategy required someone to talk to the athletes about their perceptions of the BFMP. The group concurred that I might be ideally placed to conduct such an interview. I agreed to undertake this task on behalf of the group and set about devising an interview schedule; an early draft of this was peer-reviewed within my own university department. A further draft of the schedule incorporated ideas from the practitioner group.

Phase three: Monitoring and reflecting on the views of the client group

Semi-structured interviews were conducted with injured athletes at the Centre. During the following 4 weeks, nine athletes were interviewed—seven of whom had opted to attend the body-fat, one-to-one consultation procedure, the remainder had not taken up this option. This reflected Centre records for the take-up rate, which was calculated to vary around the 80% mark. Data from this process resulted in the categories shown in Figs 10.5–10.7.

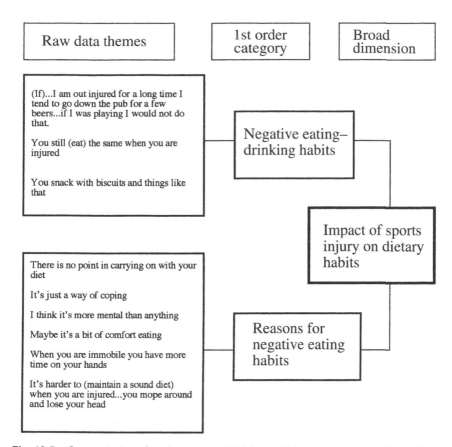

Fig. 10.5   Categorizations from interviews with injured athletes: injury and eating habits.

Summary of the interview material

A number of factors emerged from the athlete interviews. For example, a number of reasons for putting on body weight during injury were reported. In some cases, boredom was cited. Other athletes spoke of changing habits because they were not competing. Comfort eating and eating due to feelings of depression were also highlighted (see Figure 10.5). Figure 10.6 indicates that seven out of the nine athletes found the BFMP informative. The educational aspect of the procedure was also generally appreciated, and some athletes saw the one-to-one meetings as a positive learning exercise.

However, these supportive comments were not universal, and Fig. 10.7 highlights some less-favourable views. Those who chose not to attend the one-to-one meetings expected to recover in the short term (and expected increases in training activity to take care of any excess body-fat), received low body-fat readings or felt they had sufficient prior knowledge. One athlete

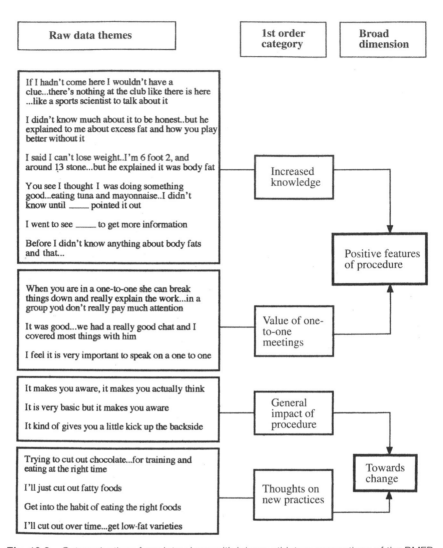

Raw data themes	1st order category	Broad dimension

If I hadn't come here I wouldn't have a clue...there's nothing at the club like there is here ...like a sports scientist to talk about it

I didn't know much about it to be honest..but he explained to me about excess fat and how you play better without it

I said I can't lose weight..I'm 6 foot 2, and around 13 stone...but he explained it was body fat

You see I thought I was doing something good...eating tuna and mayonnaise..I didn't know until _____ pointed it out

I went to see _____ to get more information

Before I didn't know anything about body fats and that...

Increased knowledge

When you are in a one-to-one she can break things down and really explain the work...in a group you don't really pay much attention

It was good...we had a really good chat and I covered most things with him

I feel it is very important to speak on a one to one

Value of one-to-one meetings

Positive features of procedure

It makes you aware, it makes you actually think

It is very basic but it makes you aware

It kind of gives you a little kick up the backside

General impact of procedure

Trying to cut out chocolate...for training and eating at the right time

I'll just cut out fatty foods

Get into the habit of eating the right foods

I'll cut out over time...get low-fat varieties

Thoughts on new practices

Towards change

Fig. 10.6   Categorizations from interviews with injures athletes: perceptions of the BMFP.

suggested that the BFMP could be improved, and indicated that a personal diet plan would help (see Fig. 10.7).

Phase four: Reflections on client data and ongoing practice

As in Phase two, the monitoring results were forwarded to the practitioner group by the outside facilitator before the next reflection meeting. The group were encouraged to propose alternative interpretations, contest any issues, or highlight alternative perspectives. The practitioners felt that the findings

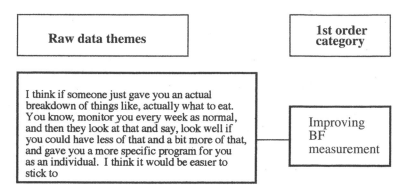

Raw data themes	1st order category

I think if someone just gave you an actual breakdown of things like, actually what to eat. You know, monitor you every week as normal, and then they look at that and say, look well if you could have less of that and a bit more of that, and gave you a more specific program for you as an individual. I think it would be easier to stick to   —   Improving BF measurement

Fig. 10.7 Categorization from interviews with injured athletes: ways to improve the program.

underscored a need for the body-fat program to be offered to other athletes and were encouraged by the positive nature of the feedback.

As in the previous meeting, it was clear that the sport scientists had been reflecting on practice since we last met. This was encouraging, and it indicated that practitioners were taking account of a variety of information. This embraced an awareness of past reflections (documented in Phase one of the project) and also included an ongoing review of current practice. At this stage, I was able to supplement this historical and current information with the feedback provided by the client group.

This array of information stimulated a lively debate during the meeting and the practitioners clearly drew from this widening body of knowledge. As an example, it was noted that injured athletes who had attended the one-to-one talks had found them to be valuable. This feedback reinforced the practitioners earlier views of ideal practice, which had highlighted the value of one-to-one meetings. However, in the minds of the sport scientists the one-to-one aspect of the body-fat procedure had recently developed into a time-based problem. This created a certain practical tension. The practitioners remained convinced that one-to-one meetings were best, but they were also becoming increasingly aware that it was a time-consuming procedure:

> ... if you see them [the injured athletes] for an hour each, you are looking at a minimum of two hours' work and you are repeating yourself at least four times. But it needs time and it needs a one-to-one ... really. (Reflection meeting: sport scientist.)

Such was the perceived pressure on time that the need to maintain a one-to-one approach was challenged:

> ... There is common stuff [to all athletes] so you could do it with two, you can talk to one and the other would listen. (Reflection meeting: sport scientist.)

However, any attempt to move away from a one-to-one process was quickly rejected:

> ... I still think one-to-one is better ... when there are two in a group, they won't ask the questions they want to ask ... what we need to do is the one-to-ones still. (Reflection meeting: sport scientist.)

As time progressed, the meeting increasingly concentrated on the detail of practice (mainly craft-based issues), and the nature of the advice that needed to be given was also discussed (a combination of craft and professional issues). As an example of this debate, one sport scientist spoke about different cases that they had encountered. Some athletes needed to lose body-fat:

> ... he had put on 10 lbs [4 kg]...he was adamant that he was fine, that there was no problem. (Reflection meeting: sport scientist.)

In contrast, others needed to eat more to assist the recovery process:

> ... he [the player] said, 'I want some advice on building myself-up'. He was eating nothing all day ... he was going to bed starving. I told him he needed to make sure he was fit and strong and that would give his knee the best chance of recovering. (Reflection meeting: sport scientist.)

The discussion focused on this issue and the practitioners began to see an argument for changing the emphasis of the body-fat procedure:

> ... we talk about it as weight and body-fat assessment ... you are looking at it as a dietary screen and a weight and body-fat assessment to check ... that the emphasis is correct ... first and foremost on their diet, to make sure they are fuelling themselves properly. (Reflection meeting: sport scientist.)

The other sport scientist felt that this was what they had always done:

> ... That is what we always try to emphasize anyway. Even when you say you have to lose some weight ... you still have to make sure that you are eating enough and you are gearing the diet to recover from the injury. (Reflection meeting: sport scientist.)

An idea was eventually floated that the one-to-one talk needed to be specific not generic and to emphasize either weight-loss or fuelling-up issues:

> The two main things here are the weight-loss issue and fuelling issue. So you have two who have weight concerns and two guys who need to make sure they maximize their potential. So you talk to the two on the weight-loss issue and off they go and the other guys, you talk to them [about weight gain]. (Reflection meeting: sport scientist.)

Again, this was not viewed as a positive move:

> I don't know because ... as they are losing weight you still want to make sure that their diet is going to be adequate, and is still going to be adequate in future to support their training ... It doesn't do them any harm to learn by both sides. I don't think it actually does them any harm to recognize that you

don't gain weight overnight and you don't lose it overnight. (Reflection meeting: sport scientist.)

This phase of the discussion ended with a commitment from the two sport scientists to ensure that the one-to-one consultation included both weight-loss and sustainable-diet information. It was also stressed that the material presented should relate to the needs of the athlete, so making the consultation less regimented and more needs-focused.

The meeting ended with a number of core decisions/suggestions being made by the practitioner group.

- Despite problems with the time-consuming nature of the one-to-one consultations, this aspect of the procedure would remain.

- The nature of the consultation would, to a large degree, be dependent on the needs of the athlete. However, all consultations would stress the core principles of a sensible diet and highlight the need to eat well to maximize performance.

- Consultation times would be clearly organized to ensure that appointment times were kept. It was hoped that this clarification would prevent athletes or sport scientists from waiting around.

Overview and practitioner conclusions

This section will present a summary of the practitioners' thoughts on what had become a 15-month project. The practitioners' underlying objective was to explore the possibility of sharing practice between the disciplines of sports science and physiotherapy. The barrier to formalizing issues in the past had been linked to limitations on the time available to talk. The practitioners all felt that the project had helped to overcome this particular barrier:

The meetings that you had with us certainly helped me to reflect in my mind about how I worked with those people...I know it is important to sit down and talk things through and how much value is placed on that...and time consuming as it is...the benefits outweigh the negatives. (Reflective interview: sports scientist.)

It helps to keep things developing...instead of just working within your own area you can keep developing certain aspects of your work and developing links between the two sides. Just this process in itself has proved to us that there is a lot we need to keep working on and improving...communicating across the group. The meetings showed us how much information we can get across to each other and sort of...the team approach to problem solving gets a whole lot more done, so problem solving together helps...what it also did as an overall process is that it identified...areas that we need to be concerned about in our working practices. It has led to a greater awareness of the need for staff training and the need to work at working practices generally. (Reflection meetings: sport scientist.)

The physiotherapist within the group also put forward his views on the structure of the meetings that had taken place. He paid particular attention to, what he saw as, the positive aspect of the facilitator's role:

I find the meetings useful ... there is a lot to be said for having someone else there who hasn't got a particular axe to grind ... and facilitates it ... acts as a sounding board ... I think you get a greater degree of balance in the debate. (Reflection meeting: physiotherapist.)

The second sport scientist agreed and also stressed the value of linking feedback on practice to the reflective process:

The real great thing about it [the reflection on the body-fat program] from our point of view was that we got a lot of positive feedback about the job we were actually doing ... we are not getting that from anywhere else and it makes it worthwhile actually doing it ... feedback whether good or bad and reflecting on what you're doing is beneficial. (Reflection interview: sport scientist.)

In conclusion, elements of this practical illustration can be linked to the literature outlined in the first section of this chapter. First of all, the project followed a pathway of formalized reflection and ongoing action. In addition, the discussion brought into play elements of craft knowledge (i.e. dealing sensitively with athletes in the one-to-one meetings and reconciling the tensions between time constraints and ideal practice). Examples of integration between craft and professional knowledge were also encountered as the nature of 'educational' input was discussed. In this case, craft knowledge was based on the experience of listening to injured athletes. In contrast, professional knowledge drew from the practitioners' understanding of the implications that accompanied different forms of dietary advice. Furthermore, the general structure of the process can be broadly aligned with the action-research cycle outlined in Fig. 10.1.

With reference to ideas presented in the second section, my role, as outsider, was multifaceted in nature. My tasks included organizing and chairing group meetings and collecting/collating information from practitioner and client sources. Finally, I should stress that the project described here was undertaken with enthusiastic, skilled, and committed sports injury practitioners. Maybe of even greater importance, they also all worked well together. In combination, these background factors allowed my involvement to develop into a rewarding and straightforward experience, for which I am extremely grateful. It is, however, unrealistic to expect all workplace settings to be so functional; and where working relationships are less harmonious, it follows that the instigation and maintenance of any reflective process may be more difficult.

References

1. Carr, W. and Kemmis, S. (1986). *Becoming critical: Education, knowledge and action research.* Falmer, London.
2. Cullen, J. (1996). Appraising teacher quality: using action research to develop a new process. *Educational Action Research,* **4**, 245–56.
3. Elliott, J. (1991). *Action research for educational change.* Open University Press, Milton Keynes, Bucks.
4. Hart, E. and Bond, M. (1995). *Action research in health and social care.* Open University Press, Milton Keynes, Bucks.
5. Lewin, K. (1946). Action research and minority problems. *Journal of Social Issues,* **2**, 34–6.
6. Tinning, R. (1992). Reading action research: Notes on knowledge and human interest. *QUEST,* **44**, 152–7.
7. Schon, D. A. (1983). *The reflective practitioner.* Basic Books, New York.
8. Schon, D. A. (1987). *Educating the reflective practitioner.* Jossey Bass, San Francisco, CA.
9. McFee. G. (1993). Reflections on the nature of action-research. *Cambridge Journal of Education,* **23**, 173–83.
10. Gilbourne, D. and Taylor, A. H. (1998). From theory to practice: The integration of goal-perspective theory and life development approaches within an injury specific goal-setting program. *Journal of Applied Sport Psychology,* **10**, 124–39.
11. Gilbourne, D., Taylor, A., Downie, G., and Newton, P. (1996). Goal-setting during sports injury rehabilitation: A presentation of underlying theory, administration procedure, and an athlete case study. *Sports Exercise and Injury,* **2**, 1–10.
12. De Guana, P. R., Diaz, C., Gonzalez, V., and Garaizar, I. (1995). Teachers' professional development as a process of critical action research. *Educational Action Research,* **3**, 183–94.
13. Titchen, A. and Binnie, A. (1993). Research partnerships: Collaborative action research in nursing. *Journal of Advanced Nursing,* **18**, 858–65.
14. Hart, E. and Bond, M. (1996). Making sense of action research through the use of a typology. *Journal of Advanced Nursing,* **23**, 153–9.
15. McTaggart, R., Henry, H., and Johnson, E. (1997). Traces of participatory action research: Reciprocity among educators. *Educational Action Research,* **5**, 123-41.
16. Stringer, E. T. (1996). *Action research: A handbook for practitioners.* Sage, London.
17. Kickett, D., McCauley, D., and Stringer, E. (1986). *Community development processes: An introductory handbook.* Curtin University of Technology, Perth, Australia.
18. Gilbourne, D. (1998). Collaborative research involving the sport psychologist within action research themes and processes. Unpublished doctoral dissertation, University of Brighton, UK.

Index